4-MINUTE WORKOUTS FOR EVERY BODY

TABATA
WORKOUT
HANDBOOK

ACHIEVE MAXIMUM FITNESS
WITH OVER 100
HIGH INTENSITY INTERVAL TRAINING
WORKOUT PLANS

ROGER HALL

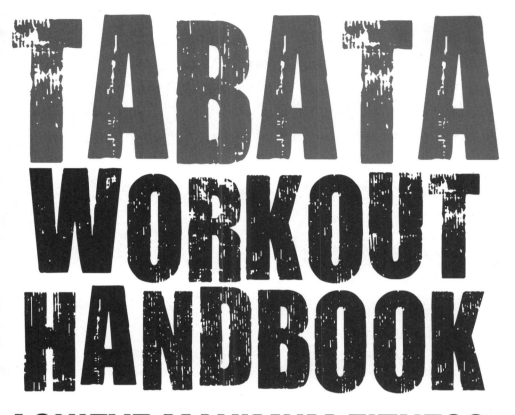

hatherleigh

Tabata Workout Handbook
Text copyright © 2015 Roger Hall

All rights reserved. No part of this book may be reproduced, stored in a retrieval system, or transmitted, in any form or by any means, electronic or otherwise, without written permission from the Publisher.

Library of Congress Cataloging-in-Publication Data is available upon request.
ISBN 978-1-57826-561-9

All Hatherleigh Press titles are available for bulk purchase, special promotions, and premiums. For information about reselling and special purchase opportunities, please call 1-800-528-2550 and ask for the Special Sales Manager.

Cover and Interior Design by Heather Magnan

10 9 8 7 6 5 4 3 2 1
Printed in the United States

CONTENTS

LET'S GET STARTED!

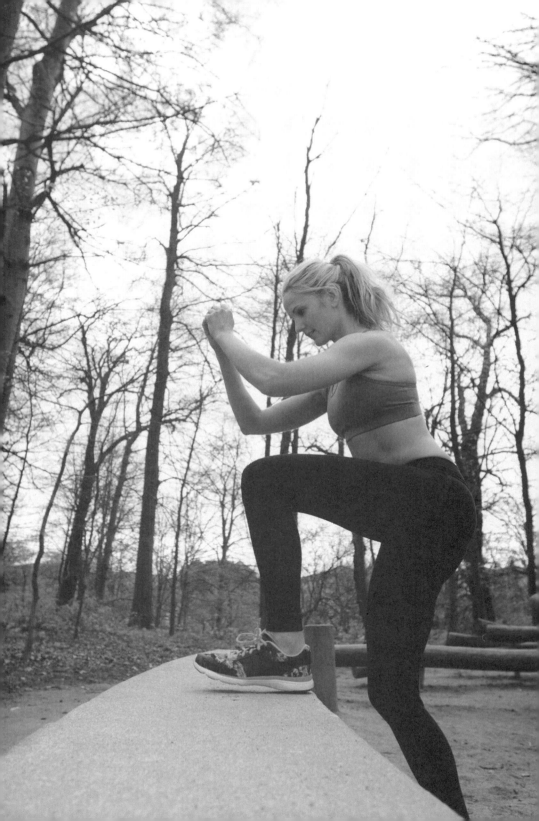

WHAT IS TABATA?

The Tabata Training Method

Designed to afford the body an efficient workout—with maximum benefits—in a short amount of time, the tabata training method uses high intensity interval training to provide a full workout, building strength and improving cardio condition. Developed and tested by esteemed physiologist Dr. Izumi Tabata in Tokyo, tabata allows for practical, reliable results even under the tight time restrictions of the modern lifestyle. At four minutes per exercise, tabata workouts can easily be completed on a lunch break!

Training tabata style allows you to shed fat while maintaining current fitness levels and building more muscle. Whether used as your primary means of working out, or as a way to simply add some extra variety and intensity to your weekly routine, tabata style training is fast, efficient, flexible, and above all—it works!

A tabata interval works as follows: Working at the maximum capacity that your body and technique allows for, exercise intensely for 20 seconds. Following this, rest for 10 seconds. Continue low-stress movement, making sure to control your breathing as you prepare to resume full-force motion. Repeat this cycle, focusing on one exercise at a time, for a total of eight intervals per exercise.

This style of training allows for tabata's integration with a wide variety of fitness programs. Applicable with or without body weights, free weights (or a combination of the two), squats, burpees, stationary and spin bikes, even sprinting are all potential avenues for tabata interval training. The primary focus is on maintaining one's top-level effort throughout the interval, and completing all eight intervals before allowing the body to fully relax.

The key to tabata training, particularly when integrating tabata into an existing workout routine, is to only use weights and movements that are appropriate (in other words, easy enough or difficult enough) for you. Remember that as you continue to work out, your body will begin to change as it improves; exercises that were once difficult will become easy! Be aware of this; as you begin to see progress, continue to advance your fitness goals, using options that are challenging to you.

Many of the workouts in this book can be completed with little to no equipment, and can be performed virtually anywhere. If you *do* have some basic equipment, integrating weights or resistance into your tabata workout can provide even more significant results.

That being said, tabata style training *is* an advanced method of working out, and may present some difficulty for the inexperienced. When working out, and especially when working out alone, it can be difficult to maintain the good form that would normally keep you safe—particularly when working out intensely. Before beginning your workout, spend about 10 minutes doing some joint mobility stretches. Practice the movements in your workout, completing between 5–10 repetitions of each, to familiarize yourself with the motions and create muscle memory for the movement as a whole.

The importance of form is paramount—not just in terms of safety, but in terms of your fitness results. When I train clients in my gym, I always encourage them to fight against the clock, not just for one more rep, but for one more rep with *perfect form*. This is more difficult to achieve, and will require you to rest more, but the best way to get strong is to complete all of your movements with excellent body mechanics. If it is a struggle for you, keep at it! In a few weeks, come back and try the same workout again; see how much progress you have made.

TRACK YOUR PROGRESS

One of the best ways to track your own progress is by "scoring" yourself. Write down the number of burpees, sit ups, or kettlebell swings you completed in your last 4 minute interval. Then, when you do the same workout again, check your new count against what you did the last time. This will let you know if you are progressing, and whether it is time to find a new variation of the movement—one that is a bit more difficult, to ensure you continue to get stronger!

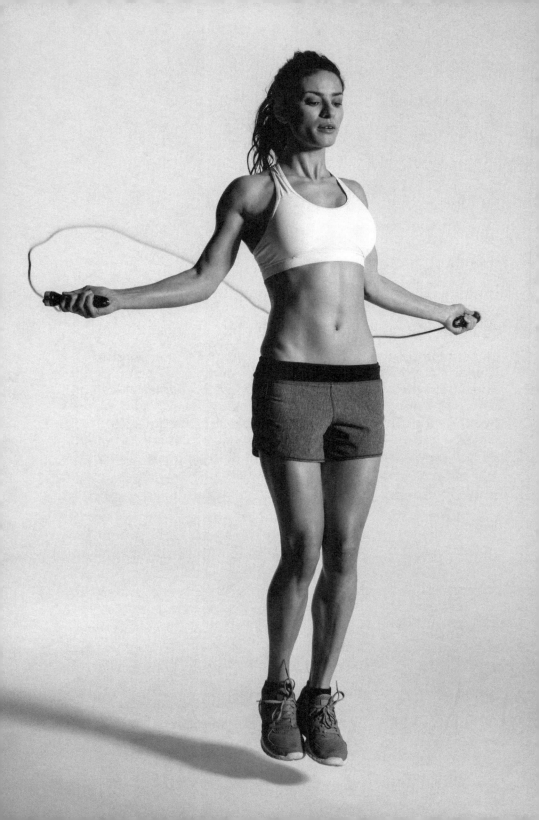

BENEFITS OF TABATA

Research has shown that exercise focused on short, intense bursts of energy where the heart rate reaches about 90 percent of its maximum capacity, interspersed with short periods of rest, is significantly more effective at increasing overall fitness levels.

Tabata training is more effective at increasing both one's VO2 max (maximal aerobic capacity) and anaerobic capacity than other forms of interval training and distance training. It also raises your metabolism and allows you to burn more body fat, letting you get much more out of your workout, all in a substantially shorter time frame. And, because the movements are so intense and always change, tabata routines remain fun and engaging.

With each workout only taking 16 minutes to complete (plus a little warm up time) tabata workouts are convenient and easy to fit into your day. They can be done whenever or wherever you like, and the movements can even be modified to fit your time, place, and overall fitness and energy levels, letting you stay safe while you work to achieve your fitness goals.

SOME BENEFITS OF TABATA TRAINING INCLUDE:

- Improved fitness level in a short amount of time
- Increased aerobic and anaerobic capacity
- More stamina
- Increased lean muscle mass
- Decreased body fat
- Better cardiorespiratory capacity
- Strength gains

Tabata training is a great fitness tool that can be used as a stand-alone training program for anyone who wants to increase their fitness levels, gain strength, and shed body fat. When exercising for these purposes, it is recommended to do tabata workouts three to four times per week, as long as you are sufficiently recovered and have rested appropriately between workouts. With this approach, tabata work combined with a healthy diet is a quick and easy way to help you build strength and lose fat.

Tabata work can also be used in conjunction with other sport-specific or goal-specific training routines to help you become faster and stronger, while increasing your capacity to work at maximum levels over a longer period of time. Using high intensity interval training is more effective, more interesting, and quicker than using running to increase cardio capacity or to trim unwanted body fat.

GENERAL TERMS AND GUIDANCE

How to Use This Book

This book can be used in a variety of different ways, depending on your fitness goals. If your goal is to increase your condition level, all while maintaining your current fitness program, tabata makes for a great supplement. If you are instead looking for a fitness plan that you can perform on your own without expensive equipment or a designated workout space, tabata provides great results with minimal investment. However, to get the most benefit possible from this handbook, you should consider investing in a few key pieces of equipment—multipurpose tools suitable for a wide range of fitness programs.

We recommend:
• A few kettlebells of differing weights (at least one you can swing and one you can put over your head)
• Dumbbells
• A pull-up bar
• Good, all-purpose athletic shoes

The key is to pick the exercises that you know you can do and complete them with higher intensity. Try to pick three to four workouts each week that target all of your major muscle groups. Following this, take a rest day; a break between tabata workouts will allow your body to recover more fully, and get stronger as a result. If you still want to work out on your off days, doing some "active recovery" exercises like biking, taking a brisk walk, or going for a light jog are all great ways of letting your body catch its breath.

As your fitness level increases, you may need to alter some of the workouts to ensure they continue to meet your needs. If you feel the need to supplement the exercises, try to maintain the basic movements themselves, and focus on increasing the movement's *difficulty*. In terms of maintaining one's form and safety while exercising, do *not* try to modify the movement itself to be more complex. You open yourself up to unnecessary risk, and there are still easier ways of increasing your workout's gain.

For example: the basic movement of a kettlebell swing is the hip hinge. If you feel that swinging the weight you have is becoming too easy, you can start to use a heavier kettlebell, try deadlifting with a heavier barbell, or try doing a snatch instead. If there is a workout that calls for a push press, but your weights are too light, try to keep within the basic "push" movement. You could perform an exercise where you push something away from your body—a strict press, a deficit push-up or a handstand push-up would all be acceptable substitutes. If air squats are too easy, turn them into front squats, or even jumping squats. Pulling movements should always be substituted for another pull. If you don't have a pull-up bar, you can clean, or do rows or snatches.

Above all, when altering a movement in this book to allow for more options or more challenge, remember the basics of the tabata interval: anything you change will still need to be realistic as a part of a tabata interval.

Your work time for each movement remains fixed at only 4 minutes. After practicing each movement between 5 to 10 times, and making sure that you are sufficiently warmed up, work as hard and as fast as you can (while maintaining good form and rhythm) for 20 seconds. Following this (and all subsequent periods of activity in the workout) rest for 10 seconds. When you rest, try to keep moving, keeping the working body parts loose and moving. Repeat this cycle eight times for a total of 4 minutes per exercise.

Helpful Terminology

Active Recovery: During your rest or recovery period, continue to move by shaking out your legs or arms to help your body pump blood and oxygen back to your fatigued muscles. You can also do some isometric holds, such as a plank pose. Performing isometric holds is also a way to increase the difficulty level of the tabata workout.

Bodyweight Movements: An exercise using only the weight of your body.

Compound Movements: An exercise that involves multiple muscle groups.

Distance Training: Training your body to run or move at a low intensity over distance for a longer period of time.

High Intensity Interval Training (HIIT): Training in short but intense bursts of energy followed by a rest period.

Interval Training: A method of training where the athlete alternates between two or more exercises.

Isometric Hold: Holding a joint and muscle group in one position.

During this type of exercise, your muscles will not lengthen and contract; they will stay the same.

Maximal Aerobic Capacity (VO$_2$ Max): The maximum amount of oxygen the body can use during a specified period of (usually) intense exercise. VO$_2$ depends on one's body weight and the strength of the lungs. Also known as maximal oxygen consumption, maximal oxygen uptake, and max VO$_2$.

Plyometric: Also known as "jump training," where the muscles are made to exert maximum force in short intervals, with the goal of increasing speed and power.

Reps (or Repetitions): The number of times you complete an exercise.

Rest: The rest or recovery phase when an athlete stops working. Keeping the rest short and the work intense will increase fitness and fat loss. During the rest period, try to stay active by moving around and shaking out tension. This will help the body recover so that you can work with intensity again.

Sets: For the purposes of this book, a set refers to completing 10 reps. Exercises will often call for a specific number of sets.

Tabata: A method of High Intensity Interval Training (HIIT) where the athlete works for 20 seconds and rests for 10 seconds, repeating eight sets usually consisting of four movements.

KEEPING TIME

Because so many of tabata's advantages depend on you keeping to a strict schedule of activity, keeping accurate time is doubly important. There are a variety of tools available to help you keep time during your workout. A clock with a second hand or any of the free timer apps available for most smartphones work perfectly well. If you're looking to spend money on a good sports timer, I recommend a Gymboss Timer. Easy to use and extremely convenient, these are small, fully programmable sports timers that can attach to your belt or sit on the floor. If you plan on incorporating a lot of tabata training or interval work into your fitness regimen, I highly suggest purchasing one.

EXERCISE DESCRIPTIONS

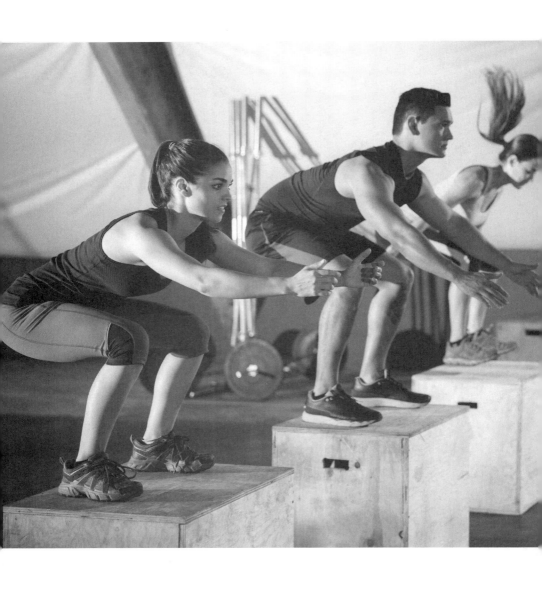

BODY WEIGHT EXERCISES

AIR SQUAT

Begin with your feet shoulder distance apart, with the toes pointing slightly away from each other. Send your hips down, and then back until your hip crease goes below your knees. Engage the glutes to stand up. During the squat, your knees should track out over your toes, but should not *pass* the toes. While squatting, try to keep the weight in the mid-foot. If squatting below parallel is difficult for you to achieve, you should regularly practice performing squats against a wall.

ALTERNATING LUNGE STEP

Lunge forward, then back. Switch legs each step. Always stay in the same place.

BEAR CRAWL

Begin on your hands and knees with your hands directly under your shoulders and the knees right under the hips. Lifting your knees to about 6 inches off the ground, step forward with the left foot, then the right hand; the right foot, and then the left hand. Stay in this position for the prescribed time or distance. Keep your hips low and your weight evenly distributed between the feet and hands.

BENCH STEP UP WITH KNEE/LEG RAISE

Stand facing a box or bench of appropriate height with the feet together. Step one leg up onto the box and fully extend that hip. As you stand up, flex at the other hip, drawing the knee up as high as you can. Reverse this movement to step down. Perform this movement holding a weight if possible.

BICYCLE CRUNCH

Lay on your back with your hands behind your head. Bring your knees up to your chest and extend one leg straight out. Keep your lower back flat on the ground. Quickly bring your right elbow to your left knee, and then alternate sides as quickly as you can.

BOTTOM TO BOTTOM SQUAT

This is performed exactly as an air squat, except that the rest portion of this movement is completed at the bottom of the squat position.

BOX JUMP (ON BENCH)/STEP-UP

From a standing position, swing your arms back, and then sweep the arms forwards, bringing both knees up and landing with your full foot on a box, bench, or other stable surface you can jump on. Stand up fully, extending the hips at the top. Either jump or step back down.

BRIDGE

Lay on your back with your feet between hip and shoulder distance apart, and your knees bent at about 45 degrees. Take a deep breath in, drive your heels into the ground, squeeze your glutes, and then send your hips towards the sky while trying to make your body into a straight line through the shoulders, hips, and knees. Keep the glutes tight, and continue to push the hips higher as your flexibility increases.

BURPEE

Stand with your feet shoulder distance apart. Fold at the waist and place hands just in front of and outside the feet. Jump or step with both feet back to the Elbow Plank position (see page 21), perform a push-up, and then jump or walk both feet up close to the hands as you send your hips straight up, and then stand up. If the push-up is too difficult, you can take it out until you develop the strength.

BURPEE BOX JUMP

Perform a burpee, but instead of jumping up and clapping above your head at the end, jump up or step up onto an appropriate size box or bench.

BURPEE LONG JUMP

Perform a burpee, but instead of jumping up and clapping above your head at the end, stand with both feet hip distance apart. Sweep your arms back, and jump as far as you can with one leap. Perform another burpee when you land.

BURPEE LUNGE STEP

Perform a burpee, but instead of jumping up and clapping above your head at the end, perform a lunge step with each leg.

BUTT KICKERS

Leaning forward, run as quickly as you can, while bringing your heels as close to your buttocks as possible.

DEAD BUG

Lay on your back with your upper and lower back pressed into the floor or mat. Extend your legs and arms and lower them as close to the ground as you can while maintaining a flat back. Raise one arm and the opposing leg slowly, and then return them to their starting position as you raise the other arm and leg.

DECLINE PUSH-UP

Perform a push-up as usual, but keep your feet elevated off the ground. The higher you can lift your feet, the more difficult the movement will be. As with all push-ups, keep the abs, glutes and quads engaged to be sure you use your core.

DEFICIT PUSH-UP

Perform a push-up with your hands elevated on two stable surfaces, which allows for a deeper range of motion. You can use yoga blocks, two even-sized kettlebells, or two same sized dumbbells. To make this movement more difficult, elevate your feet on a stable surface.

DIAMOND PUSH-UP

Perform a push-up as usual, save that your hands should be positioned under the sternum, with the index fingers and thumbs touching, in the shape of a diamond. Touch your chest to your hands with every repetition.

DIP

Situate a chair in a way that it will not move (you may also use a couch or any other stable piece of furniture). Stand in front of the chair with your hands firmly planted on the seat behind you, below your shoulders. Lower yourself until your shoulders dip below your elbows and your arms are at 90 degree angles. You may support yourself with your feet on the other chair until you become strong enough to perform this movement without assistance.

You may also sit on the floor with your feet flat on the ground, knees bent, and your buttocks lifted off the ground. Lower your body down until your buttocks touches the ground, and then press back up.

If you are in a traditional gym setting that has a dip machine, set the machine to the appropriate height (low enough to use your feet for assistance should you need to, or high enough so that your feet do not touch the ground, if you do not need assistance). Beginning with both arms locked out and your shoulders back, lower your body down until your elbows are at a 90 degree angle or less, then press back up. Try to keep your feet pointed at the ground.

Variations of this exercise include: the Couch Dip, Floor Dip, Triceps Dip and Elevated Dip.

ELBOW PLANK

Begin by lying face down with your elbows directly under or slightly in front of your shoulders (your hands may be clasped together or slightly apart). Lift your hips so that your shoulders, hips, knees, and ankles are in a straight line. Tuck your tailbone towards your nose to make your back flat. Tighten the quads and glutes, and pull your elbows towards your toes, as if trying to fold your body in half, but don't let your body move. Drive the balls of your feet into the ground. Maintain body tension while breathing. The plank may also be performed on the hands, a variation which will be referred to in this handbook as the Tall Plank. The difference between the two movements is that, in the Tall Plank position, the hands are directly under the shoulders. Think of the Tall Plank as the "top" of the Push-Up and Mountain Climbers motions.

FLUTTER KICK

Lay on your back with your hands placed under your lower glutes, keeping the tailbone elevated. Keep your feet 3 to 6 inches off the ground. Repeatedly raise one foot about 6 inches and lower the other.

GRAPEVINE OR KARAOKE STEP

With your arms straight out to the sides, cross your left foot over the right, stepping out with the right, and then cross the left foot behind the right, stepping out with the right. Continue moving to the side, and then repeat by leading with the opposite foot. This movement opens and stretches the hips and helps increase agility and speed.

HAND RELEASE PUSH-UP

Perform a push-up as usual, but at the bottom of the push-up, when your chest touches the ground, lift both hands off the ground. Do not worm at all on the way up; keep the movement completely strict, using your arms and core to lift your body off the ground.

HANDSTAND HOLD

Place your hands firmly on the floor, about shoulder distance apart, with your fingertips spread apart. Walk your feet towards your hands until you are in a triangular position. Stretch one leg up towards the ceiling behind you and try to kick off with the other, only going as far as you are comfortable in this position. If you feel okay with kicking your feet over your head, continue to kick up until you are in a full handstand position with your back to the wall. Try to maintain the same body position as when you are in the Elbow Plank (see page 21), with the tailbone tucked and the abs and glutes engaged. Performing a proper handstand is a combination of both balance and strength.

HANDSTAND PUSH-UP

There are many variations of handstand push-ups. A basic way to get started is to place a very firm mat or cushion under where your head will touch to protect your head and neck. This movement should only be done with complete control and consideration for your safety. If done incorrectly, this movement can cause severe neck injury. Begin in the handstand position; lower your head towards the mat so that it comes into contact as the top of a three-point triangle with your hands. Touch the top of your head to the mat, and then push back up with your arms. You can begin practicing this movement by lowering yourself as far as you can with control then pushing back up. Gradually, your strength will increase and you will be able to achieve a full handstand push-up.

HIGH KNEES

Hold your hands at waist height or higher. Taking short, quick steps, pump your knee to your hand and then quickly repeat on the other side. The focus of high knees should be on taking a lot of very quick steps in a short distance, not on taking a few steps over a long distance.

HOLLOW BODY

Lay on your back with your hands extended behind your head. With your arms fully extended behind you, grab an anchor, like a heavy kettlebell or a piece of furniture that will not move. Lift your legs straight up in the air, pressing your upper and lower back flat on the ground, and slowly lower your feet, maintaining the position of your back. Keep your legs as low as possible and your upper and lower back flat to the ground. Start to press the hands into the anchor as though you were trying to lift it straight up to the ceiling, but do not move it. This will engage your arms, lats and upper abdominals, making the movement more difficult.

HOLLOW BODY LEG LIFT

Once you achieve the hollow body position (see page 23), slowly raise and lower your legs.

JUMPING LUNGE

From the bottom of the lunge position, jump with both legs and land in the lunge position with the opposite leg forward. At the top of this movement, both legs should be straight, causing you to jump higher, instead of keeping your legs bent and not jumping very high (which will be easier, but not very effective).

JUMPING SQUAT/JUMPING AIR SQUAT

Stand with feet shoulder distance apart with the toes pointed slightly out. Pull the hips down and back until the hip crease is below the knee. Launch yourself into the air, fully opening your hips at the top of the movement. Land with feet shoulder distance apart, resetting the feet if needed, and repeat. Be sure to keep the knees tracking *out* over the toes. If you ever have knee pain during this movement, switch to regular air squats.

LONG JUMP

With your feet hip distance apart, swing your way back, and then sweep them forward as you jump as far as you can while landing with your feet out in front of you.

L-SIT

Place two stable, non-slip chairs facing together. Place your hands on the chairs, with your hands under your shoulders, and in line with your hips. Begin by lifting the knees up and feet off the ground, then attempt to straighten the legs. Try to keep your hips in line or slightly behind your arms. If you cannot get your legs straight, keep trying! Just keep the knees as high as possible and keep trying to straighten the legs. As you get stronger, this will improve.

LUNGE

Stand with feet hip distance apart. Take a big step forward with one foot and plant the front foot firmly on the ground. Lower your body, touching your back knee to the ground (if you are able). Keep your front knee over the ankle at all times. Press your body off the ground with the front foot and bring both feet together. Repeat on both sides for one repetition. If you want to do this with weights, you can hold one in front of your chest, or two in either hand.

MOUNTAIN CLIMBER/GRASS HOPPER

Begin in the Tall Plank position (see page 21) with your hands directly under your shoulders, with the shoulders, hips, and ankles all in a straight line. Bring your left knee to the outside of your left elbow if your flexibility allows for it (if not, bring it as close to the elbow as possible). Then, launch both legs in the air to switch positions, landing with your right knee outside your right elbow.

Increase or decrease the intensity of this movement by performing the movement quickly or slowly. For an additional challenge, you can try Grasshoppers, which are performed similarly to the Mountain Climber, but instead of touching your knee to the elbow on the same side you bring the knee under the belly and touch it to the opposite elbow.

ONE-LEG BRIDGE

While in the bridge position, lift one foot off the ground and point it straight up to the ceiling. Keep the opposite foot flat on the ground. Alternate sides each interval.

ONE-LEG PUSH-UP

Perform push-ups as normal, but with only one leg on the ground. This will target the core and abdominals more than a traditional push-up.

PLANK-UP

From an Elbow Plank position (see page 21), place one hand flat on the ground, then the other hand flat on the ground, and fully extend both arms. Lower yourself back to Elbow Plank position in the same way you got up.

PLANK WALK OUT

Assume the top of a push-up position with your hands directly under your shoulders, and your ears, shoulders, hips, knees and ankles in a straight line. If this is already difficult, you may stop here. To proceed: maintaining your body in this position, take small steps with your hands in front of your body. Get as low as you can by walking your hands straight out in front of you while maintaining a neutral back position. You should not have any lower back pain. If you do, it means that you lowered your hips and are not maintaining a neutral spine.

PLYO PUSH-UP

Perform a push-up as usual, but outside your hands should be two even blocks, or raised platforms that are totally stable. Note that the higher the height of the blocks, the more difficult the movement. When performing the push-up, explode from the bottom of the push-up and land with both hands on top of the raised platforms, instead of on the ground. This should be an explosive jumping movement with your hands, not a step. Walk or jump your hands back down to the ground, and repeat.

POWER SKIP

Skip the same way you did as a kid, but with each stride bring your knee as high into the air as you can, utilizing a pumping motion with the opposite arm to propel your body as vertically as you can.

PUSH-UP

Begin in the Tall Plank position (see page 21) with your hands aligned directly under your shoulders, fingertips pointed away from each other. The shoulders, hips, knees and ankles should all be in a straight line. As you initiate the descent, the elbows should travel backwards, with the upper arms staying as close to the body as possible.

Maintain full core tension for the entire time you are descending. Your body should travel downwards until your arms are at 90 degree angles, or until your chest touches the ground. If at any time you lose core tension and are unable to maintain the straight line through the shoulder, hip, and ankle line, you have gone too deep into the movement.

REVERSE LUNGE

Lunge one leg back behind your body, and then step forward. These are much more stable than forward lunges, as your center of gravity does not change (as it does with other lunge steps). You may hold a weight for an additional challenge.

REVERSE SIT UP

Laying flat on your back, bring your knees up so your thighs are at 90 degrees to your torso and fully extend your legs over your hips. Raise your hips off the ground as if you are trying to touch the ceiling above you with your toes. Lower your hips back to the ground with control.

RUN BACKWARDS

Running backwards is exactly as it sounds. It helps improve coordination and agility, uses your normal running muscles differently, and forces your foot to strike the ground in a different manner. If you are nervous about running backwards, begin by running backwards up a hill. This will force you to run slower and increase your confidence in this movement. Plus, if you trip and fall backwards, you will be closer to the ground.

SIDE PLANK

Begin in the Elbow Plank position (see page 21) but lift your left arm off the ground, until your torso and hips are at a 90 degree angle to the ground. Extend your left arm towards the ceiling. If this is difficult, you can take your left leg and place it either in front of or behind the other leg.

SIT UP

Lay on your back with your knees butterflied out and the bottoms of your feet touching. Hold a kettlebell upside down and by the horns in front of your chest. Sit up until your shoulder passes the hip crease.

SPIDERMAN CRAWL

Begin on your hands and knees and lift your knees about 6 inches off the ground. Keeping the hips low, step forward at the same time with one hand and the opposite leg and do a push-up getting your chest as low to the ground as possible. Push back up, and then step forward with the other hand and opposite foot. Continue to walk forward in this fashion.

SPIDERMAN PLANK

Begin in either the Elbow Plank or the Tall Plank position (see page 21). With a neutral spine (no arch in the low back, keeping the tailbone tucked) bring your knee to your elbow or the upper arm, and push the knee into the arm as hard as you can before returning the leg behind the body. Repeat on the other side. If you cannot reach your knee to your elbow, get it as close as you can.

SPLIT SQUAT

This exercise can be performed with a weight, but try it without a weight first to test your strength and ability during this movement. Stand with your feet together, and then jump one leg forward and one leg back, flexing at the knees and lowering your hips. Do not allow your knee to crash into the ground (although it may gently touch the ground if you can control the movement). Immediately reverse the movement, switching the position of your legs. You may return to standing in between. To make the movement more difficult, your legs should be straight at the top of the switch, without touching the ground.

SPRINT

Run as fast as you can. As you fatigue, your pace will slow, but try to hit your top speed at your current fatigue level each time.

SQUAT JACK

Stand with your feet together, and your hands behind your head. Send your hips back as you jump your feet out to about shoulder distance apart, and then jump your feet back together and stand up completely.

SQUAT THRUST

Begin in a standing position. Bend at the waist and place both hands on the ground, directly under your shoulders. Kick both legs back, so that your body is in a straight line going from the shoulder, through the hips and ankles. Jump or walk your feet back up outside your hands and stand up completely.

STEP UP

From a standing position, flex at the hip, bringing one foot up on the box or bench. Stand up, fully extending the hips at the top. Step back down and repeat with the other leg.

SUPERMAN

Lie on your stomach with your arms fully extended in front of you, while simultaneously raising your upper torso and your thighs off the ground. Keep your shoulders pulled down and back while fully engaging your glutes. If you cannot raise the shoulders and the thighs at the same time, first raise the shoulders, and then raise the thighs. Eventually you will develop the strength and flexibility to raise both simultaneously.

TAPPING PLANK

From an Elbow Plank position (see page 21), reach out in front you fully extending your arm to touch a target at least forearms distance away from you.

TUCK JUMP

Begin with your feet hip distance apart, holding your hands in front of you at about waist height. Bend at the knees and dip down slightly, driving your feet off the ground and up towards your hands. Try to touch your knees to your hands. Re-extend your legs and land on the balls of your feet. Make certain to absorb the shock of the landing by bending your knees. Try to keep your weight in the balls of your feet; do not slam your heels into the ground.

The Tuck Jump is meant to serve as a substitution for jumping rope. You may jump rope in any place where this book calls for Tuck Jumps.

UPHILL SPRINT

Sprint up a hill as fast as you can (the steeper, the better). If you do not have a hill available, you can run up stairs or simply sprint on flat ground.

V-UP

Lie flat on your back with your arms and legs extended. Keeping your buttocks on the ground, touch your fingers to your toes by folding your body in half at the waist. If this is too difficult, begin by touching your knees, then ankles, and toes when it becomes easier.

WALKING LUNGE

Take continuous forward lunge steps, alternating sides each step. You may hold a weight for an extra challenge.

YOGA PUSH-UP

Begin by lying on the ground with your hands under your shoulders and your feet hip distance apart. Push up off the ground and establish a strong Tall Plank position (see page 21) with your ears, shoulders, hips, and ankles all in a straight line. Pull your chest back towards your knees, creating a triangle position with your body. Looking straight ahead or slightly up, send your chest towards the ground with a scooping motion, keeping your hips elevated. As your chest gets closer to the ground, bring your hips in line with your shoulders and ankles, and then lie on the ground. Point the toes back and press your upper body up, keeping your shoulders back and using the traps to keep your chest up. Lower your torso back to the ground, take a deep breath in, and press back up into the Tall Plank.

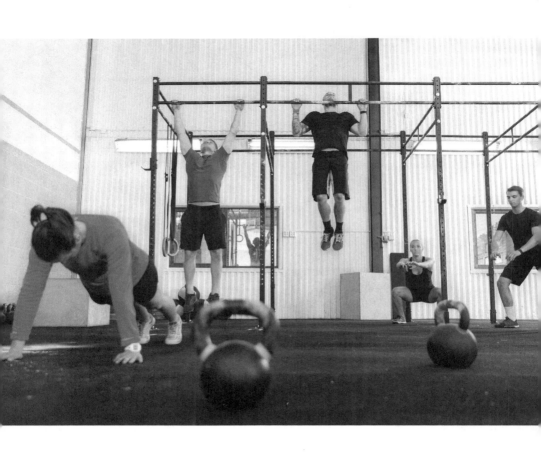

MINIMAL GEAR EXERCISES

BENT OVER ROW

Stand with feet hip to shoulder distance apart. Bend at the waist, maintaining a flat (neutral) back position. Hold two dumbbells directly under your shoulders. Keeping your shoulders down and back and your eyes straight ahead, row the dumbbells up until they get as close to your chest as possible. Slowly return them to the starting position.

DUMBBELL BENCH PRESS

Lie on a flat bench with dumbbells resting in your hands on your thighs. Use your legs to help bring the dumbbells right next to your shoulders with palms facing forward, away from your body. Take a deep breath in and breathe out as you use your chest to press the dumbbells overhead, until you achieve full lockout of your arms. Breathe in as you lower the dumbbells back to the starting position.

DUMBBELL FLY

Lie on a flat bench with a dumbbell in each hand and resting on your thighs. Use your thighs to help raise the dumbbells over your shoulders, but keep your arms slightly bent. Lower the dumbbells away from each other as you breathe in. When you feel a stretch in your chest, breathe out and return the dumbbells to the starting position. Try to maintain the same angle in your arms throughout the movement.

DUMBBELL HANG CLEAN

For the Dumbbell Hang Clean, the dumbbells are hanging at your sides in either hand. Bend at the knees and hinge your hips, driving the dumbbells up to the rack position (see page 43). Hold the dumbbells in the rack during the rest period.

DUMBBELL SUMO SQUAT

Hold a dumbbell at the base with your arms straight. Your legs should be wider than shoulder distance apart with the toes pointed away from each other at an angle. Your arms should not move during this exercise. As you breathe in, bend at the knees, sending the hips back and down until your thighs are parallel to the floor. Breathe out as you stand up, squeezing the glutes and abs and driving through the heels as you return to your starting position. You should maintain perfect posture and a neutral spine during all parts of this movement.

FORWARD LUNGE WITH TWO DUMBBELLS

Performed the same as a reverse lunge (see page 36) but step your working leg forward instead of backwards.

JUMP ROPE

Hold a properly sized jump rope (when you step on the rope with one foot, both handles should reach up to your armpits) in each hand. Swing the rope over your head and jump over it. A very efficient way to do this is to keep your hands at waist height and spin the rope using only the momentum from the wrists.

LATERAL RAISE

Pick up a pair of dumbbells and stand with torso vertical, with the arms slightly bent and the palms facing in. Without swinging the dumbbells, and with hands tilted slightly forward, lift the dumbbells until your arms are parallel to the floor. Lower the dumbbells back to the starting position. You may perform this standing or seated. Always choose a weight that allows you to maintain proper form.

OVERHEAD WALKING LUNGE

Hold a dumbbell (or a plate or kettlebell) over your head with two hands and lunge forward, alternating legs each step.

PULL-UP

With your palms facing away from the body, grab a pull-up bar with your hands (about shoulder distance apart). Hang from the bar, staying active in the shoulder girdle. Pull yourself up towards the bar until your chest almost touches the bar. Maintain a neutral body position throughout this movement, engaging the abs, glutes and quads the entire time. There are many variations of the pull-up, so feel free to experiment.

REVERSE LUNGE WITH WEIGHTS

Stand holding a pair of dumbbells with your feet together. Keep your shoulders back and down and your head up. Take a step backward with one leg, landing the ball of your foot on the ground, bending both knees and lowering your back knee to the floor (if you can do it with control). If not, stop before you lose control. Stand back up, driving through the mid-foot and heel of your front leg and the ball of the foot of your back leg. Return to a standing position and do the same thing on the opposite leg. For the safety of your knee, the knee of the front leg should stay over the ankle, and should never track out past the toes and should not fall inward. If this happens to you, try to lighten up the weight or use no weights at all.

SEATED BICEP CURL

Sit on the edge of a flat bench with a dumbbell in each hand and the arms fully extended, with your palms facing your body. Maintaining little to no movement in the upper arms, curl the arms up, turning the palms away from each other as you do then slowly return the dumbbells to the starting position.

SHOULDER PRESS

This movement may be performed either seated or standing, and can utilize dumbbells (or other weights such as barbells or kettle-bells). Dumbbells and kettlebells allow for a more natural shoulder position.
From a standing position with dumbbells, stand with your feet under your hips and the dumbbells next to your shoulders with the hands facing forward. Take a deep breath in, engage the quads, glutes and abdominals, and press the dumbbells straight up until they touch at the top. Lower the dumbbells down, maintaining control the entire time.

WEIGHTED LUNGE

Hold dumbbells (or kettlebells) in the rack position (see page 43) or at your sides and lunge forward or backwards.

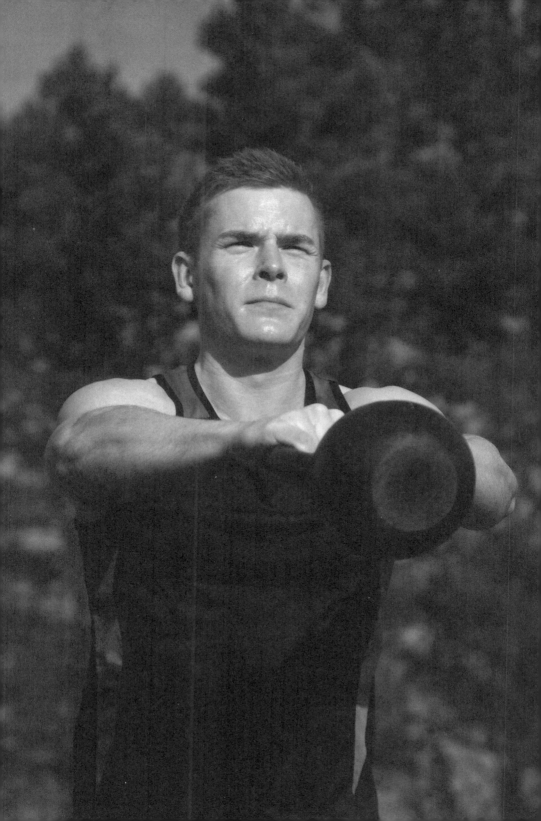

KETTLEBELL EXERCISES

KB CLEAN

Hold one or two kettlebells. Starting from the rack position (see page 43), hike the kettlebell back between your legs, loading up the hamstrings and glutes. Then, drive your hips forward and bring the kettlebell in the straightest line possible, back to the rack position. If you use two kettlebells, hike both back between the legs at the same time. With dumbbells, touch the bell to the floor and use the hips to drive the bell back up to the rack position.

KB CLEAN AND PRESS

Perform a Clean (see above), followed by a Strict Press (see page 42).

KB CLEAN AND PUSH PRESS

Perform a Clean (see above), followed by a Push Press (see page 42).

KB CLEAN AND THRUSTER

Perform a Clean (see page 39), and then perform a Thruster (see page 45).

KB DEAD LIFT

Stand with your feet shoulder distance apart, with the kettlebell handle centered between your heels. Hinge at the hips, keeping your weight in your heels. Your shoulders should stay back, with the neck and spine in a neutral position, always looking straight ahead, not up or down. Grab the kettlebell with both hands, keeping the arms straight. Breathe in through the nose, tightening the abs and glutes to create tension through your whole body. Squeeze your glutes and drive through your heels. Fully extend your hips and keep your abs, glutes, and quads tight. Stand up straight at the top, and do not lean back. Descend by hinging at the hips, sending the hips back. Bend your knees and lower the kettlebell back to the floor between your feet.

KB FRONT SQUAT

Hold one or two kettlebells in the rack position (see page 43). Stand with feet between hip and shoulder distance apart. Take a deep breath in, then bend your knees and send your hips slightly down, then back. Continue to send the hips down and back until your hip crease goes below the knee. Keep your shoulders back and chest up. The knees should track out over the toes, but not go out past the toes.

KB GOBLET SQUAT

Hold a kettlebell by the sides of the handles (by the "horns") and stand with your feet approximately shoulder distance apart, with toes pointed slightly away from each other. Take a deep breath in, hold your breath, and firm up your abs. Send your hips down and then back until your hip crease goes below parallel. Your back should maintain a neutral position, not rounding in the lower back as you reach the bottom of this position. If you cannot achieve this position, do not squat as low and work on hip mobility until you can achieve this position safely.

KB HANG CLEAN

This is performed exactly the same as a kettlebell or dumbbell Clean, but the kettlebell is cleaned from a dead hang position half-way between the knee and ankle; there is no extra backswing. Use only your hips to drive the kettlebell up from a stationary position.

KB ONE-LEG DEAD LIFT

The One-Leg Dead Lift can be performed by holding one kettlebell in front of you with both hands, or with two kettlebells at your sides (with one kettlebell in each hand).

When using one kettlebell, begin with the big toe of your working leg pointed directly at the kettlebell. The toe or shoe may be touching the kettlebell; just be careful when setting the kettlebell back down!

When using two kettlebells, begin with the center of the handles in line with your mid-foot. Stand tall with your shoulders back. Hinge at the hips, sending them back as with the regular Dead Lift (see page 40). However, send your non-working foot back as you fold at the hips and bend at the working knee. Throughout the movement, the hips should remain level; do not lift the hip of the non-working leg.

Continue to bend at the knee and send your buttocks back until you establish a grip on the kettlebell (or kettlebells). Take a sharp breath in through the nose, tighten the abs, and lift the kettlebell(s) from the ground using the glutes of the working leg. At the top of the lift, your quads, glutes, and abs should be tight, with the shoulders back and down. Descend to the ground by sending the hips back, bending at the knee, and return the kettlebell(s) to the exact same spot they started in.

KB POWER SWING

Begin as with a regular KB Two-Handed Swing (see page 44). Hike the kettlebell back between your legs until your forearms touch your inner thighs. Drive through the heels, and stand up, launching the kettlebell to chest height, and then back between the legs again until the forearms touch the inner thighs, and back again to touch the floor in front of you.

KB PRESS/STRICT PRESS/OVERHEAD PRESS

Hold one or two kettlebells in the rack position (see page 43). Take a sharp breath in through the nose, engaging the quads, glutes, and abs (for full body tension). Squeeze the kettlebell tight and make a fist with your resting hand (which will help to engage all of the upper body muscles necessary for this movement). Slowly press the kettlebell slightly out on a diagonal, then up until your arm reaches full extension. The arm should be locked out and the shoulder packed and down, creating space between your bicep and ear. After reaching the top, the kettlebell should be stable and not wobbling around. Keep the body tight, then slowly lower the kettlebell back down to the rack position.

KB PUSH PRESS

Hold one or two kettlebells in the rack position (see page 43). Take a sharp breath in through the nose. Slightly bend at the knees, quickly dipping the body down with torso upright, and then immediately drive through the heels and extend the hips, using the legs to drive the kettlebell overhead. Use the abs and glutes for this movement by strongly engaging them as you extend the hips.

After locking out the kettlebell, lower the weight back to the rack position. Take another deep breath in and repeat as necessary.

KB RACK HOLD (RACK POSITION)

Hold one or two kettlebells or dumbbells in your hands just under shoulder level, with your wrists straight and elbows tight to the rib cage. With kettlebells, the ball part of the bell should be resting on your wrist and upper pectorals; for women, the wrist may be farther away from the chest for comfort and safety.

This is the position from which you should press.

KB RENEGADE ROW

Place two kettlebells of the same weight shoulder distance apart. Begin in a Tall Plank position (see page 21) with your hands on the kettlebells. Row one kettlebell to the chest, then the other. Rowing once on the left and once on the right constitutes one rep. To make this movement easier, place your resting hand on the floor instead of the other kettlebell.

KB RUSSIAN TWIST

Sit on the floor with your knees bent. Hold the kettlebell by the horns in front of your chest. Rotate your shoulders and torso to the left, as though crunching the right shoulder to the left hip. Bring the kettlebell and torso back to the center, and then rotate to the right, touching the kettlebell to the ground on both sides of the body. Touching the kettlebell to the ground once on the left and once on the right constitutes one rep.

To increase the difficulty of this movement, elevate your feet off the ground.

KB SNATCH

Begin as with a regular One-Handed Swing (see below). Use a very forceful hip thrust to hike the kettlebell up. When the kettlebell reaches about belly button height, begin to abbreviate the arc of the swing by pulling the elbow high and to the outside, as with the One-Hand High Pull. Punch through the handle so the kettlebell lands on the back of your wrist. When all of the timing works perfectly, the kettlebell should land on your wrist at the exact same moment that your arm locks out over your head. At the top of the movement, the shoulder is packed, and the bicep is *next* to the ear, not behind. The wrist should be straight.

To send the kettlebell down, relax and bend the arm, allowing the kettlebell to roll off the wrist. At about belly button height, hike the kettlebell back strongly, sending the hips back. This is especially important with the Snatch because a strong backswing allows you to recruit the glutes and hamstrings. Use a very strong hip snap on the next rep.

Be sure to breathe out strongly when you open the hips to power the kettlebell up into the top of the movement. The Snatch is an all-over body movement, but the engine (as with most of the swing movements) is the hips!

KB SWING

Begin with your feet approximately shoulder distance apart with the toes pointing slightly out. The kettlebells should be about 8 to 12 inches in front of your toes. With your shoulders back and down, hinge at the hips, as you send your arms down and back.

Reach out and grab the kettlebell handle with two hands. In this position, your knees should be directly over your ankles, which should create tension in your hamstrings and glutes. This action will "load" these muscle groups, getting them ready to fire. Take a sharp breath in through the nose; hike the kettlebell back between your legs with your lat muscles, until your forearms touch your inner thighs. Immediately snap the hips forward by tightening the abs, glutes, and quads, fully opening the hips at the top of the swing. As the gravity of the kettlebell begins to take it back down, engage your lats to speed up the kettlebell as it continues towards your hips. When your upper arms touch the rib cage (the kettlebell will be close to the hips at this time), hinge at the hips, sending the hips backward, and the kettlebell back above your knees (never below the knees). When you reach the end of the backswing, drive the kettlebell through the legs again and fully extend the hips to complete the second swing, launching the kettlebell forward and up again, using the power of your leg, hip, and abdominal muscles.

The kettlebell swing can be performed with one hand as well. The one-handed swing is performed in exactly the same way as the two-handed swing, but using only one hand. When you hike the kettlebell back between your legs, the "resting" arm should mimic this pattern, sweeping away from and behind your body. As the kettlebell swings up, this hand should travel in the same direction as the kettlebell and will meet the "working" hand at the top of the swing. This will help you keep your shoulders square at the top of the swing and will give you something to do with your resting hand.

KB THRUSTER

The Thruster is a powerful, all-over body movement that is a combination of a KB Front Squat (see page 40) and a KB Push Press (see page 42). It should be performed with the same hip speed of the KB Swing; but, instead of a front-to-back movement of the hips, you drive the hips straight up to launch the kettlebell overhead.

Begin with one or two kettlebells in the rack position (see page 43) and lower yourself to the bottom of the KB Front Squat. At the bottom of the squat, begin accelerating the hips straight up. Drive through the heels, forcefully engaging the abdominals and the glutes, and launch the kettlebell(s) straight overhead by transferring the speed of the hips into the kettlebell(s). End at the top of the Push Press position (see page 42), with the kettlebells stable and the shoulders packed.

If you find you are leaning back at the top of this movement or are experiencing lower back pain, the kettlebells you are using are too heavy. Try to keep the abs tighter, or lower the weight of the kettlebells if you need to. As your strength and technique develops, you will increase the weight and speed of the movement. Do not let your heels come off the ground.

KB TWO-HAND HIGH PULL

The KB Two-Hand High Pull is executed exactly as the Two-Handed Swing (see page 44), but on the upswing, when the kettlebell reaches the belt level, pull the kettlebell in with two hands, sending the elbows out and high. The hands should touch or come close to touching the chest at sternum level. Punch the kettlebell quickly out and down back where it came from, then hike the kettlebell back between the knees as with the backswing of the regular Two-Handed Swing. Be sure to maintain a firm grip on the kettlebell during this movement; do not let the kettlebell flip up and hit you in the face!

KB WIDE LEG DEAD LIFT

Begin with a loaded bar or kettlebell on the floor in front of you. Pull the bar to your shins (almost touching) or bring the kettlebell centered between your mid-foot to heel. Hinge at the hips and grip the bar directly below your shoulders. At the bottom of the movement keep your shoulders back, head and neck neutral with the eyes looking straight ahead. To stand up, take a deep breath in. As you breathe out, drive through the heels, engage the hamstrings, glutes, and abdominals, and fully extend the hips. Return the weight to the ground by hinging at the hips and controlling the weight all the way down.

GYM EXERCISES

BACK EXTENSION

On the Back Extension machine, with your ankles under the foot pads and upper thighs across the wide pad, bend at the waist, keeping your body straight. There should be no rounding of the back. You may hold a plate if you would like extra resistance. Bend forward as far as you can while maintaining a neutral lower back until you feel a stretch in your hamstrings, and then raise your torso back up to your beginning position. To avoid injury, do not round your back at any time for this movement, even to get increased range of motion.

BARBELL BACK SQUAT

Use a squat rack (adjusted to the proper height) and place a weight that is appropriate for about 10 to 15 repetitions (a relatively light weight) on the bar. Step under the bar and place the bar on your back so that it rests on your trapezius muscles. Place both hands on the bar in a position that is comfortable for your shoulders. Your wrists should be straight, and both your thumbs and fingers should be on *top* of the bar. This will keep you safe in case you need to release the bar mid-squat. Your feet should be about shoulder distance apart with the toes pointed slightly out. Take a deep belly breath in and hold it. Lower your hips and send them backwards, maintaining a flat lower back at the bottom of the squat position. You can check this using a mirror, smartphone with video recorder, or by asking a friend or trainer. You should at least break parallel if your mobility allows for it. Breathe out and engage the glutes and abdominals to stand up.

BARBELL HANG CLEANS

Dead lift a loaded barbell and stand up straight. This is the hang position. From here, quickly send the hips back, and then drive them forward as you shrug both shoulders up to your ears. Driving your hips forward into the barbell, pull it up quickly with the elbows high and outside, and then dip your body down and send your elbows forward to catch the barbell in the rack position (see page 43). As the barbell lands close to the collar bones, slightly loosen your grip on the bar, as it is difficult for some people to achieve this position with a tight grip.

HANG CLEAN WITH BARBELL

Stand with feet shoulder width apart with an overhand grip on a barbell and a neutral spine. Bend at the knees and hips and explosively extend (open) the hips, shrugging your shoulders up towards your ears. When your hips are fully open, shrug your shoulders and flex your arms quickly, driving the elbows up and forward. Receive the bar in the front squat position. Depending on how hard you drive with the hips, the depth of the squat may vary, but you will have to get as low as you need to in order to catch the bar. Stand up with your core engaged and elbows up. Lower the bar back to the hang position and repeat. This is *not* a bicep curl; it should use more leg drive than arm pull. When you transition from the hanging position to the rack, you will have to loosen your grip on the bar to allow it to slide through your hands.

INCLINE PRESS

Sit on an incline bench with two dumbbells resting on your thighs. Use your legs to help push the bells into position over your shoulders, with your palms facing away from your body. Take a deep breath in, and then breathe out as you press the bells straight up, achieving full lockout at the top of the movement. With control, lower the weights back down to your chest. For safety purposes, do not drop the dumbbells; lower them first to your thighs, and then to the ground.

LATERAL JUMP

Stand next to a cone, hurdle, barbell, dumbbell, kettlebell or other object of appropriate height. Standing on either one leg or two, hop sideways over the object, and then immediately hop back to the starting position. If using one leg, remember to alternate with each round.

LAT PULL DOWN (NARROW GRIP)

Use the same bar and technique as with the Lat Pull Down (Wide Grip) (see below), but your hands should be placed at closer than shoulder distance.

LAT PULL DOWN (WIDE GRIP)

Sit at the Pull-Down machine with the wide bar attached to the pulley. Be sure the machine fits your body. Grab the bar at wider than shoulder distance. With your chest up and shoulders back and down, pull the bar down until it touches your upper chest. Your torso should not move as you pull the bar towards it.

LEG CURL

Adjust the Leg Curl machine so it fits your body; the pads should be around your ankles. Holding the support handles, breathe out as you lift the pads, flexing at the knee, lifting the pads as close to your buttocks as possible. Lower the leg while maintaining control over the weight.

LEG PRESS WITH TOES OUT

On a Leg Press machine, place your legs on the platform at about shoulder distance apart with the toes pointed out at an angle. Hold the platform in place as you lower the safety bars and fully extend your legs without completely locking out the knees. Your torso should be at a 90 degree angle to your legs. Breathing in, lower the platform until your knees are bent at a 90 degree angle, then push with your heels and extend your legs. Lock the safety pins once completed. Take every safety precaution to avoid injury.

ONE-LEG SQUAT (PISTOL SQUAT)

If you find that you can do many two-leg body weight squats in a row, you may want to attempt a one-leg, or pistol squat. As simple as it sounds, it is very difficult. Stand on one foot, reach one leg in the air, send your hips back and down until your hip creases go below parallel, and then stand back up. Repeat on the other side. To work up to this, try the following variations. For each of these variations, be sure to breathe when you stand up and use your ab-dominals!

On a bench: Standing in front of a bench, control your hips as you lower them down, and then raise your body back up. Continue to lower the bench until you can do this without assistance.

Assisted pistol: Use any sturdy vertical object or gymnastics rings to control your descent and ascent.

Weighted pistol: Hold a small weight in front of you to help maintain balance as you lower and raise yourself.

REAR DELTOID FLY

Adjust the Cable machine so that the pulleys are above your head. Grab the left pulley with your right hand and the right pulley with your left hand so that the cables cross in front of you. Move your arms back and away from each other, keeping the arms as straight as possible.

ROMAN CHAIR KNEE/LEG RAISE

Get into the chair so that your forearms are on the pads, with your hands gripping the handles and your back against the rest. Take your feet off the rests so that they are hanging straight down, and then lift your knees as high as possible, pressing your lower back against the rest. To make this more difficult, you can perform Roman Chair leg raises, where one raises their fully extended legs as high as possible before returning to a hanging position.

SIDE SQUAT

Rest a barbell below your neck on the trapezius muscles and place your hands over the bar, slightly wider than shoulder distance, or where it is comfortable. Place your feet wide apart with the foot of the lead leg angled out to the side. Lower your body towards the lead leg as you hinge at the hip and bend the knee, keeping the other leg slightly bent. Breathe in as you lower your body and breathe out as you stand up to full hip extension of the lead leg.

SKULL CRUSHER (WITH ELASTIC BAND, DUMBBELL, BARBELL, OR EZ CURL BAR)

With a curl bar, use a narrow grip. Lie on a flat or decline bench and lower the weight over your head while keeping your elbows pointed at the ceiling. Lower the bar until it almost touches your forehead. Then with an explosive movement, push the bar up to full lockout of the elbows. As with any movement, begin with a very light weight that you can control.

STANDING BICEP CURL

Stand upright, holding the barbell at about shoulder distance with your palms facing away from your body. Maintain little to no movement in your body as you contract your biceps. Breathe out, and bring the bar towards your shoulders until the biceps are fully contracted. Slowly lower the bar to starting position.

SUMO DEAD LIFT

With your feet wider than shoulder distance and toes pointed slightly out, roll a loaded barbell against your shins. Without rounding through the low back, hinge at the hips, bend at the knees and grab the barbell at about shoulder distance apart. Drive through the heels, thrust the hips forward, and stand up quickly in one motion as you breathe out. Pause at the top with the abs and glutes engaged, and then lower the bar back to starting position.

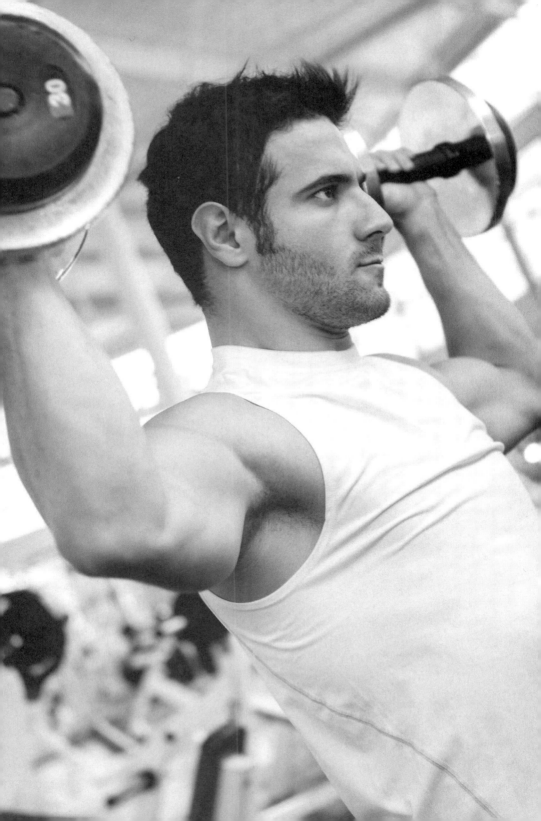

TABATA WORKOUTS

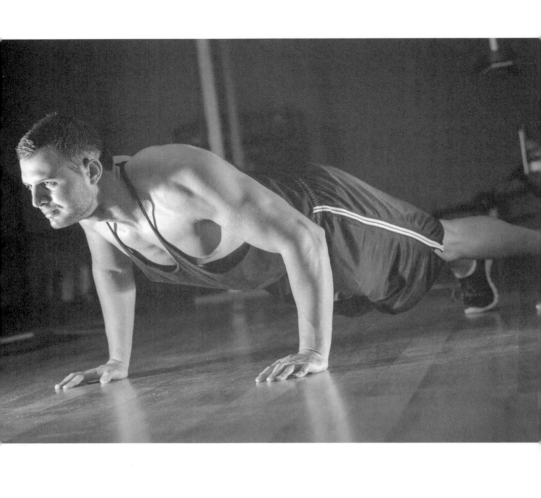

A TABATA INTERVAL WORKS AS FOLLOWS:

Working at the maximum capacity that your body and technique allow, exercise intensely for 20 seconds. Following this, rest for 10 seconds of continuous, low-stress movement, making sure to control your breathing as you prepare to resume full-force motion. Repeat this cycle, focusing on one exercise at a time, for a total of eight intervals per exercise.

The workouts in this book are generally organized with the beginner workouts, or those requiring the least amount of skill, towards the beginning of each section. Many of the workouts will focus on one or two muscle groups, but will use compound movements to do so. This means that even though you are focusing on a few muscle systems, you are still getting a full-body workout.

Some workouts are designed to work the whole body, while others focus more on one area, such as the arms, back, legs, or core. Using compound body movements makes you stronger all over and allows many body parts to work together at one time. You can select full-body workouts, or you can target specific body parts by choosing workouts that work your goal areas.

When substituting movements to make your workout harder or easier, always choose a movement that fits your ability and fitness level. For example, if you want to try a workout that has burpees but you do not feel strong with your push-ups, try substituting either push-ups or squat thrusts for that movement. You can even alternate back and forth between the two movements for the eight intervals to practice both parts of the exercise. If one of the workouts has push-ups, but they are too easy, try substituting with Deficit Push-Ups, Plyo Push-Ups, Diamond Push-Ups, or Handstand Push-Ups.

Try to make sure that you always substitute a pushing movement for another push, a pulling movement for another pull, a hinging movement for another hinge, and a squat for another squat. For example, if you do not have a pull-up bar at home, you can switch pull-ups for another pulling movement like renegade rows, heavy cleans, or even snatches, which also target the muscles of the arm and upper back. This is important because including all of these movements into your regular workouts will create balanced strength throughout your entire body and will eliminate the weakness that creeps in when workouts are not balanced.

BEGINNING TABATAS

Tabata workouts can be very intense, and therefore most are *not* suitable for the beginner fitness practitioner. However, if you are a beginner to exercise and fitness, there are many ways to make tabata workouts accessible to you.

Tabata is effective because it makes you do a lot of work in a short amount of time, with very little rest. Pay close attention to the guidance provided below and follow the beginner workouts in this section. These workouts will target your entire body and will help prepare you for the other workouts in this book. Remember, change the time and regulate your intensity by changing the volume of repetitions and the amount of weight that you use.

Always warm up first: I recommend performing 5 to 8 minutes of joint mobility exercises, followed by 10 to 20 repetitions of each movement. Arm circles, hip circles, knee circles and some light stretching should get you ready to move. After that, you can begin with a few slow repetitions of each movement. If that feels good and you feel able to perform the movement well, try to increase the pace. If you feel tightness or weakness, try to stretch that area of your body a little more or substitute the movement for something similar.

Change the time: Instead of working intensely for 20 seconds and then resting for 10 seconds, when you first start out, try working for 30 seconds and then resting for 30 seconds, and repeat each movement four times instead of eight times. As you become stronger and more able to perform each movement, try to first increase the intensity by increasing your repetitions during the work phase. Then, as you feel more comfortable with each movement, you may start working towards the 20/10 protocol.

Keep to your skill level: As a trainer, I often see people in the gym who want to perform a very high skilled movement (like the Snatch or Clean) before they have the skills needed to perform the movement perfectly. If you do not have a coach working with you, be sure to read the instructions for each movement and follow them carefully. Exercises should always be performed with high-quality movement, because if they are performed improperly it can eventually lead to injury, which will slow down your progress more than performing an "easier" or more appropriate exercise would.

Tabata #1

Squat Thrust
Air Squat
Sit Up
Push-Up

Working at maximum capacity, exercise intensely for 20 seconds. Rest for 10 seconds. Repeat each exercise interval 8 times before moving to the next exercise in the workout.

Tabata #2

Elbow Plank
KB Swing
Air Squat
KB Press

Workout Notes
**For KB Press, use 1 kettlebell or dumbbell
and alternate sides each round.**

Working at maximum capacity, exercise intensely for 20
seconds. Rest for 10 seconds. Repeat each exercise interval 8
times before moving to the next exercise in the workout.

Tabata #3

KB Goblet Squat
Push-Up
KB Swing
Tall Plank

Working at maximum capacity, exercise intensely for 20 seconds. Rest for 10 seconds. Repeat each exercise interval 8 times before moving to the next exercise in the workout.

Tabata #4

Bear Crawl
Air Squat
Push-Up
KB Press

Workout Notes
For KB Press, use 1 kettlebell or
dumbbell and alternate sides each round.

Working at maximum capacity, exercise intensely for 20
seconds. Rest for 10 seconds. Repeat each exercise interval 8
times before moving to the next exercise in the workout.

Tabata #5

KB Dead Lift
Squat Thrust
Bridge
Elbow Plank

Workout Notes
For KB Dead lift, use a light weight and focus on form.

Working at maximum capacity, exercise intensely for 20 seconds. Rest for 10 seconds. Repeat each exercise interval 8 times before moving to the next exercise in the workout.

Tabata #6

Bent Over Row
Plank
Air Squat
Bear Crawl

Working at maximum capacity, exercise intensely for 20 seconds. Rest for 10 seconds. Repeat each exercise interval 8 times before moving to the next exercise in the workout.

Tabata #7

Push-Up
Lat Pull Down
Sit-Up
Back Extension

Working at maximum capacity, exercise intensely for 20 seconds. Rest for 10 seconds. Repeat each exercise interval 8 times before moving to the next exercise in the workout.

Tabata #8

KB Swing
KB Russian Twist
KB Goblet Squat
Spiderman Plank

Working at maximum capacity, exercise intensely for 20 seconds. Rest for 10 seconds. Repeat each exercise interval 8 times before moving to the next exercise in the workout.

Tabata #9

KB Dead Lift

KB Renegade Row

Mountain Climber

Step-Up or Box Jump

Working at maximum capacity, exercise intensely for 20 seconds. Rest for 10 seconds. Repeat each exercise interval 8 times before moving to the next exercise in the workout.

Tabata #10

Squat Thrust
Sit-Up
Lunge
Plank-Up

Workout Notes
For Lunge, alternate sides each repetition.

Working at maximum capacity, exercise intensely for 20 seconds. Rest for 10 seconds. Repeat each exercise interval 8 times before moving to the next exercise in the workout.

BODY WEIGHT TABATAS

This collection of workouts is composed of routines that you can perform using only your own body weight and your environment. These workouts will increase your strength, stamina and conditioning, particularly if you are new to working out. Many of them work your entire body, helping you to lose weight while preparing to take your fitness to the next level.

Be sure to warm up properly before each workout. Body weight movements can be very difficult, especially if you choose a variation that is inappropriate for you and your fitness level. Always trust what your body is telling you, and don't work out above your own level of ability. See page 57 for more information on tailoring these and other workouts to your personal level of fitness.

Tabata #11

Push-Up
Jumping Squat
Hollow Body
Bear Crawl

Workout Notes
For Push-Up, you can also substitute it
with Plyo Push-Up. For Bear Crawl, you can
also substitute it with Spiderman Crawl.

Working at maximum capacity, exercise intensely for 20
seconds. Rest for 10 seconds. Repeat each exercise interval 8
times before moving to the next exercise in the workout.

Tabata #12

Sit Up
Bear Crawl
Handstand Push-Up
Air Squat

Workout Notes
For Handstand Push-Up, you can also substitute it with Handstand Hold.

Working at maximum capacity, exercise intensely for 20 seconds. Rest for 10 seconds. Repeat each exercise interval 8 times before moving to the next exercise in the workout.

Tabata #13

Tuck Jump
Air Squat
Elbow Plank
Lunge

Workout Notes
For Air Squat, spend any rest time
in the bottom of the squat position.

Working at maximum capacity, exercise intensely for 20
seconds. Rest for 10 seconds. Repeat each exercise interval 8
times before moving to the next exercise in the workout.

Tabata #14

Elbow Plank
Side Plank (right side)
Yoga Push-Up
Side Plank (left side)

Working at maximum capacity, exercise intensely for 20 seconds. Rest for 10 seconds. Repeat each exercise interval 8 times before moving to the next exercise in the workout.

Tabata #15

KB Russian Twist
Hollow Body
Handstand Hold
Uphill Sprint

Workout Notes
For Uphill Sprint, if you don't
have a hill, substitute Sprint.

Working at maximum capacity, exercise intensely for 20
seconds. Rest for 10 seconds. Repeat each exercise interval 8
times before moving to the next exercise in the workout.

Tabata #16

Burpee
Sit Up
Air Squat
Push-Up

Workout Notes
**For Air Squat, spend any rest time
in the bottom of the squat position.**

Working at maximum capacity, exercise intensely for 20
seconds. Rest for 10 seconds. Repeat each exercise interval 8
times before moving to the next exercise in the workout.

Tabata #17

Plank-Up
Hollow Body
Tapping Plank
Side Plank

Workout Notes
For Side Plank, alternate sides each round.

Working at maximum capacity, exercise intensely for 20 seconds. Rest for 10 seconds. Repeat each exercise interval 8 times before moving to the next exercise in the workout.

Tabata #18

Triceps Dip
Bear Crawl
Superman
Plyo Push-Up

Workout Notes
For Triceps Dip, use a couch, the floor, or dip bars.

Working at maximum capacity, exercise intensely for 20 seconds. Rest for 10 seconds. Repeat each exercise interval 8 times before moving to the next exercise in the workout.

Tabata #19

Squat Thrust
Sprint
Alt. Lunge Step
Sprint

Workout Notes
For Alternating Lunge Step, hold something heavy like a backpack full of books if Lunges are easy for you.

Working at maximum capacity, exercise intensely for 20 seconds. Rest for 10 seconds. Repeat each exercise interval 8 times before moving to the next exercise in the workout.

Tabata #20

Flutter Kick

Hollow Body

Grass Hopper

KB Russian Twist

Working at maximum capacity, exercise intensely for 20 seconds. Rest for 10 seconds. Repeat each exercise interval 8 times before moving to the next exercise in the workout.

Tabata #21

Long Jump
Air Squat
Tuck Jump
Mountain Climber

Workout Notes
For Air Squat, spend any rest time in
the bottom of the squat position.

Working at maximum capacity, exercise intensely for 20
seconds. Rest for 10 seconds. Repeat each exercise interval 8
times before moving to the next exercise in the workout.

Tabata #22

Jumping Squat
Burpee Box Jump
High Knees
Tuck Jump

Workout Notes
For Burpee Box Jump, use a bench or any stable non-slip surface. You can also substitute burpees with a very high jump at the end.

Working at maximum capacity, exercise intensely for 20 seconds. Rest for 10 seconds. Repeat each exercise interval 8 times before moving to the next exercise in the workout.

Tabata #23

Bear Crawl
Bridge
L-Sit
Plank-Up

Workout Notes
For L-Sits, use a couch.

Working at maximum capacity, exercise intensely for 20 seconds. Rest for 10 seconds. Repeat each exercise interval 8 times before moving to the next exercise in the workout.

Tabata #24

Spiderman Crawl
Air Squats
Push-Up
High Knees

Workout Notes

For Air Squat, spend any rest time in the bottom of the squat position, keeping your hands off of your legs.

Working at maximum capacity, exercise intensely for 20 seconds. Rest for 10 seconds. Repeat each exercise interval 8 times before moving to the next exercise in the workout.

Tabata #25

Walking Lunge
KB Russian Twist
Mountain Climber
One-Leg Plank

Workout Notes
For Walking Lunge, hold something heavy if Lunges are easy for you. For One-Leg Plank, alternate legs each 20 second interval.

Working at maximum capacity, exercise intensely for 20 seconds. Rest for 10 seconds. Repeat each exercise interval 8 times before moving to the next exercise in the workout.

Tabata #26

Burpee
Jumping Squat
Tapping Plank
Push-Up

Working at maximum capacity, exercise intensely for 20 seconds. Rest for 10 seconds. Repeat each exercise interval 8 times before moving to the next exercise in the workout.

Tabata #27

Sprint
Push-Up
Air Squat
Burpee

Workout Notes
For Air Squat, spend any rest time
in the bottom of the squat position.

Working at maximum capacity, exercise intensely for 20 seconds. Rest for 10 seconds. Repeat each exercise interval 8 times before moving to the next exercise in the workout.

Tabata #28

Jumping Lunge
Air Squat
Hollow Body
Bear Crawl

Workout Notes
For Air Squat, spend any rest time
in the bottom of the squat position.

Working at maximum capacity, exercise intensely for 20
seconds. Rest for 10 seconds. Repeat each exercise interval 8
times before moving to the next exercise in the workout.

Tabata #29

One-Leg Bridge
Spiderman Crawl
V-Up
Handstand Hold

Workout Notes
For One-Leg Bridge, alternate sides every interval.

Working at maximum capacity, exercise intensely for 20 seconds. Rest for 10 seconds. Repeat each exercise interval 8 times before moving to the next exercise in the workout.

Tabata #30

Elbow Plank
Mountain Climber
Push-Up
Burpee

Working at maximum capacity, exercise intensely for 20 seconds. Rest for 10 seconds. Repeat each exercise interval 8 times before moving to the next exercise in the workout.

Tabata #31

One-Leg Squat
One-Leg Push-Up
Hollow Body
Sit Up

Workout Notes
For One-Leg Squat and One-Leg Push-Up,
alternate sides each round.

Working at maximum capacity, exercise intensely for 20 seconds. Rest for 10 seconds. Repeat each exercise interval 8 times before moving to the next exercise in the workout.

Tabata #32

Sprint
Superman
Jumping Squat
Bear Crawl

Working at maximum capacity, exercise intensely for 20 seconds. Rest for 10 seconds. Repeat each exercise interval 8 times before moving to the next exercise in the workout.

Tabata #33

Dead Bug
Bicycle Crunches
Hollow Body
Elbow Plank

Working at maximum capacity, exercise intensely for 20 seconds. Rest for 10 seconds. Repeat each exercise interval 8 times before moving to the next exercise in the workout.

Tabata #34

Reverse Sit Up
Spiderman Plank
Bridge
V-Up

Workout Notes
**If Bridge is easy, try to spend
any rest time in the Plank position.**

Working at maximum capacity, exercise intensely for 20
seconds. Rest for 10 seconds. Repeat each exercise interval 8
times before moving to the next exercise in the workout.

Tabata #35

Dip
Push-Up
Superman
Plank Walk Out

Workout Notes
For Dip, use a couch or the floor.

Working at maximum capacity, exercise intensely for 20 seconds. Rest for 10 seconds. Repeat each exercise interval 8 times before moving to the next exercise in the workout.

Tabata #36

Yoga Push-Up
Elbow Plank
One-Leg Bridge
Air Squat

Workout Notes
For One-Leg Bridge, alternate sides each round.
For Air Squat, spend any rest time in the bottom
of the squat position.

Working at maximum capacity, exercise intensely for 20
seconds. Rest for 10 seconds. Repeat each exercise interval 8
times before moving to the next exercise in the workout.

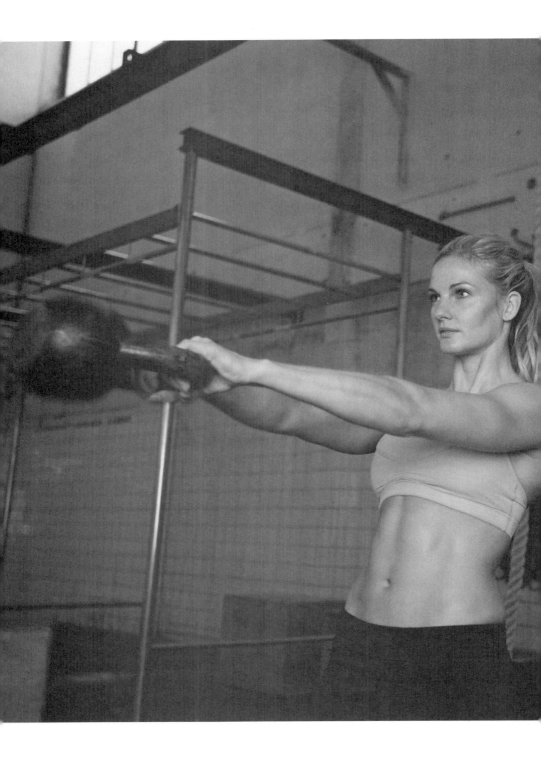

TABATAS WITH MINIMAL GEAR AND KETTLEBELLS

This section was designed for those with a few pieces of equipment available, or who are willing to invest in weights or other fitness tools. Note that even a small investment in quality equipment will result in a huge pay-off.

In this section, exercises will routinely call for kettlebells (preferable for their versatility and portability), dumbbells, or a barbell (if you have it). While a barbell is the least portable and versatile of the suggested equipment, it is easier to change the weight, which makes it more suitable than kettlebells or dumbbells for certain exercises. For more advanced practitioners this may be preferable, but for those just starting out, a few carefully selected kettlebells or dumbbells will be perfect for the majority of these routines.

To practice all of the movements in this section, you will need at least a pull-up bar, one heavy kettlebell, and two light kettlebells. The light kettlebells should be of the same weight and have flat bottoms, as you will be using them to plank, perform push-ups and rows. Bells with seams or rough bottom surfaces will make this very difficult, so avoid these. Hex dumbbells also work great for these movements, if you already have them around.

Introducing weights and more advanced body weight movements like pull-ups into your workout routine will increase your strength and fat loss exponentially. When you increase strength and muscle, your body naturally begins to burn more calories. Be sure that you practice each movement with good form several times before beginning your workouts, to ensure that you are comfortable and familiar with all parts of the routine. This becomes much more important as you add heavier weights to your exercises.

Tabata #37

Pull-Up
KB Swing
Push-Up
Burpee

Working at maximum capacity, exercise intensely for 20 seconds. Rest for 10 seconds. Repeat each exercise interval 8 times before moving to the next exercise in the workout.

Tabata #38

KB Push Press

KB Thruster

KB Front Squat

KB Thruster

Workout Notes
For KB Thruster, use two kettlebells
or a barbell and maintain the same
number of reps as the previous round.

Working at maximum capacity, exercise intensely for 20
seconds. Rest for 10 seconds. Repeat each exercise interval 8
times before moving to the next exercise in the workout.

Tabata #39

KB Strict Press

KB Front Squat

KB Renegade Row

KB Push Press

Workout Notes

For KB Strict Press, KB Front Squat, and KB Push Press, use two kettlebells. For KB Renegade Row, alternate sides every repetition.

Working at maximum capacity, exercise intensely for 20 seconds. Rest for 10 seconds. Repeat each exercise interval 8 times before moving to the next exercise in the workout.

Tabata #40

KB Swing
Jumping Squat
KB Swing
Jumping Squat

Working at maximum capacity, exercise intensely for 20 seconds. Rest for 10 seconds. Repeat each exercise interval 8 times before moving to the next exercise in the workout.

Tabata #41

Push-Up
Weighted Lunge
KB Power Swing
Burpee

Workout Notes
For Weighted Lunge, alternate legs every repetition.

Working at maximum capacity, exercise intensely for 20 seconds. Rest for 10 seconds. Repeat each exercise interval 8 times before moving to the next exercise in the workout.

Tabata #42

KB Power Swing
KB Swing
KB Two-Hand High Pull
KB Snatch

Workout Notes
For KB Snatch, you can also substitute it with One-Hand Swing and use two kettlebells.

Working at maximum capacity, exercise intensely for 20 seconds. Rest for 10 seconds. Repeat each exercise interval 8 times before moving to the next exercise in the workout.

Tabata #43

KB Dead Lift
KB Swing
Plank
KB One-Leg Dead Lift

Workout Notes
For KB One-Leg Dead Lift, use one light kettlebell and alternate legs each round.

Working at maximum capacity, exercise intensely for 20 seconds. Rest for 10 seconds. Repeat each exercise interval 8 times before moving to the next exercise in the workout.

Tabata #44

Kettlebell Swing

Deficit Push-Up

KB Front Squat

KB Renegade Row

Workout Notes

Perform the Deficit Push-Ups with your hands on two equal weighted kettlebells or dumbbells. For KB Renegade Row, alternate arms each repetition.

Working at maximum capacity, exercise intensely for 20 seconds. Rest for 10 seconds. Repeat each exercise interval 8 times before moving to the next exercise in the workout.

Tabata #45

Bent Over Row
KB Swing
KB Clean
KB Press

Workout Notes

For Bent Over Row, use two dumbbells. Perform KB Swing with one arm and alternate sides each round. For KB Clean and KB Press, alternate sides each tabata round.

Working at maximum capacity, exercise intensely for 20 seconds. Rest for 10 seconds. Repeat each exercise interval 8 times before moving to the next exercise in the workout.

Tabata #46

KB Clean & Press
KB Snatch
KB Swing
KB Front Squat

Workout Notes
For KB Clean and Press, KB Snatch, and KB
Front Squat, alternate sides each round.

Working at maximum capacity, exercise intensely for 20
seconds. Rest for 10 seconds. Repeat each exercise interval 8
times before moving to the next exercise in the workout.

Tabata #47

KB Strict Press

KB Rack Hold

KB Push Press

KB Rack Hold

Workout Notes
For KB Strict Press, alternate sides each round. For KB Rack Hold and KB Push Press, use two kettlebells

Working at maximum capacity, exercise intensely for 20 seconds. Rest for 10 seconds. Repeat each exercise interval 8 times before moving to the next exercise in the workout.

Tabata #48

Push-Up
Pull-Up
Bottom to Bottom Squat
Elbow Plank

Workout Notes
For Bottom to Bottom Squat, spend any rest time in the bottom of the squat position.

Working at maximum capacity, exercise intensely for 20 seconds. Rest for 10 seconds. Repeat each exercise interval 8 times before moving to the next exercise in the workout.

Tabata #49

KB Snatch
Sit Up
KB Strict Press
Hollow Body Leg Lift

Workout Notes
For KB Snatch, alternate sides each round.
For KB Strict Press, use two kettlebells.

Working at maximum capacity, exercise intensely for 20 seconds. Rest for 10 seconds. Repeat each exercise interval 8 times before moving to the next exercise in the workout.

Tabata #50

Burpee
KB Swing
Push-Up
KB Snatch

Workout Notes
For KB Snatch, alternate sides each round.

Working at maximum capacity, exercise intensely for 20 seconds. Rest for 10 seconds. Repeat each exercise interval 8 times before moving to the next exercise in the workout.

Tabata #51

Jump Rope
Push-Up
Mountain Climber
KB Goblet Squat

Workout Notes
For KB Goblet Squat, hold one kettlebell in front of your chest.

Working at maximum capacity, exercise intensely for 20 seconds. Rest for 10 seconds. Repeat each exercise interval 8 times before moving to the next exercise in the workout.

Tabata #52

KB Clean & Press
KB Front Squat
KB Swing
Elbow Plank

Workout Notes

For KB Clean and Press, use one kettlebell and alternate sides each round. For KB Front Squat, use the same kettlebell as with the Clean and Press.

Working at maximum capacity, exercise intensely for 20 seconds. Rest for 10 seconds. Repeat each exercise interval 8 times before moving to the next exercise in the workout.

Tabata #53

Handstand Hold
Pull-Up
Sit Up
Hollow Body

Working at maximum capacity, exercise intensely for 20 seconds. Rest for 10 seconds. Repeat each exercise interval 8 times before moving to the next exercise in the workout.

Tabata #54

Dip
KB Renegade Row
Reverse Sit Up
Dead Bug

Workout Notes
For KB Renegade Row, alternate sides each round.

Working at maximum capacity, exercise intensely for 20 seconds. Rest for 10 seconds. Repeat each exercise interval 8 times before moving to the next exercise in the workout.

Tabata #55

KB Swing
KB Dead Lift
Bicycle Crunch
KB Push Press

Workout Notes

For KB Swing, use one arm and alternate sides each round. For KB Push Press, use two kettlebells or alternate sides each interval.

Working at maximum capacity, exercise intensely for 20 seconds. Rest for 10 seconds. Repeat each exercise interval 8 times before moving to the next exercise in the workout.

Tabata #56

KB Clean
KB Push Press
KB Front Squat
Plank

Workout Notes
For KB Clean, KB Push Press, and KB Front Squat, use two kettlebells.

Working at maximum capacity, exercise intensely for 20 seconds. Rest for 10 seconds. Repeat each exercise interval 8 times before moving to the next exercise in the workout.

Tabata #57

KB Swing
Alternating Swing
Jumping Squat
Burpee

Workout Notes
For KB Swing and Alternating Swing, use one kettlebell.

Working at maximum capacity, exercise intensely for 20 seconds. Rest for 10 seconds. Repeat each exercise interval 8 times before moving to the next exercise in the workout.

Tabata #58

KB Snatch
Side Plank
Push-Up
Squat Thrust

Workout Notes
For KB Snatch and Side Plank, alternate sides each round. For Squat Thrust, move as fast as possible.

Working at maximum capacity, exercise intensely for 20 seconds. Rest for 10 seconds. Repeat each exercise interval 8 times before moving to the next exercise in the workout.

Tabata #59

Bear Crawl
Walking Lunge
Handstand Hold
Dead Bug

Working at maximum capacity, exercise intensely for 20 seconds. Rest for 10 seconds. Repeat each exercise interval 8 times before moving to the next exercise in the workout.

Tabata #60

KB Clean & Push Press
Elbow Plank
Bottom to Bottom Air Squat
One-Leg Bridge

Workout Notes

For KB Clean and Push Press, use two kettlebells or if using one kettlebell, alternate sides each interval. For One-Leg Bridge, alternate legs each interval or use both legs if you have trouble with this.

Working at maximum capacity, exercise intensely for 20 seconds. Rest for 10 seconds. Repeat each exercise interval 8 times before moving to the next exercise in the workout.

Tabata #61

KB Swing
KB Goblet Squat
Jump Rope
Push-Up

Working at maximum capacity, exercise intensely for 20 seconds. Rest for 10 seconds. Repeat each exercise interval 8 times before moving to the next exercise in the workout.

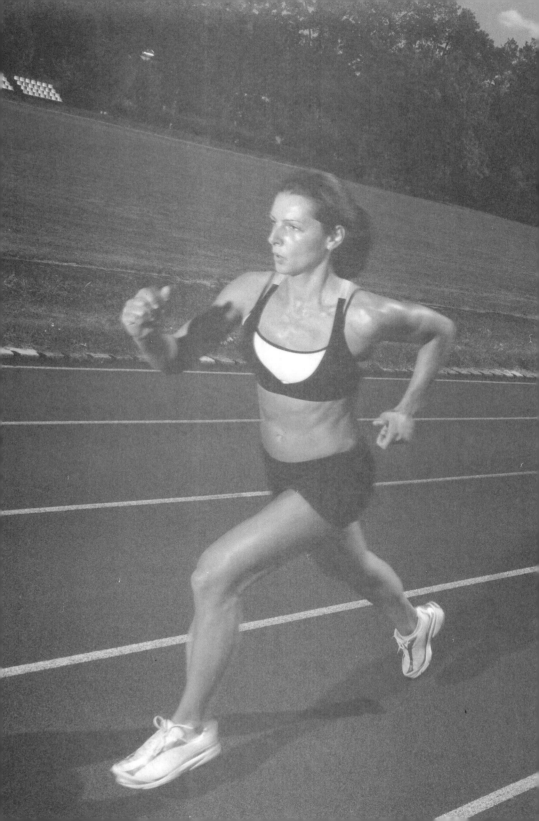

TRACK AND FIELD TABATAS

Track and field tabatas are workouts that can be completed most conveniently at a track facility. However, many of these routines can easily be accomplished wherever there is space available; they do not require a measured track. Some of the workouts do require minimal equipment, such as a medium to heavy kettlebell for basic swings or squats, and a lighter kettlebell or dumbbell for thrusters and overhead movements. Some of the workouts utilize your surroundings; for example, a bench for step-ups or box jumps or a long set of stadium stairs for running. You will also need a stopwatch or timer to help you to time your intervals correctly.

These workouts will increase your speed, stamina, agility and core strength. Feel free to change up the workouts to fit your environment, but try to maintain the concept of each movement. If there is a plyometric (jumping) movement like the long jump, but you do not have space available to jump very far, substitute a box jump or a jumping squat, to ensure your muscles are being worked in a similar way. If the workout you chose has a grapevine, but you are limited by space, substitute in high knee steps instead.

Tabata #62

Burpee
Sprint
Air Squat
Bear Crawl

Working at maximum capacity, exercise intensely for 20 seconds. Rest for 10 seconds. Repeat each exercise interval 8 times before moving to the next exercise in the workout.

Tabata #63

KB Thruster Sprint KB Thruster Sprint

Workout Notes
For KB Thruster, use two kettlebells.

Working at maximum capacity, exercise intensely for 20 seconds. Rest for 10 seconds. Repeat each exercise interval 8 times before moving to the next exercise in the workout.

Tabata #64

Run Backwards
Grapevine
Long Jump
Sprint

Working at maximum capacity, exercise intensely for 20 seconds. Rest for 10 seconds. Repeat each exercise interval 8 times before moving to the next exercise in the workout.

Tabata #65

Walking Lunge

Push-Up or Plyo-Push-Up

Box Jump

Burpee Long Jump

Workout Notes
**For Walking Lunge, hold a
weight for added difficulty.**

Working at maximum capacity, exercise intensely for 20
seconds. Rest for 10 seconds. Repeat each exercise interval 8
times before moving to the next exercise in the workout.

Tabata #66

High Knees
Sprint
Burpee
Run Backwards

Working at maximum capacity, exercise intensely for 20 seconds. Rest for 10 seconds. Repeat each exercise interval 8 times before moving to the next exercise in the workout.

Tabata #67

KB Swing
Sprint
Air Squat
Spiderman Crawl

Working at maximum capacity, exercise intensely for 20 seconds. Rest for 10 seconds. Repeat each exercise interval 8 times before moving to the next exercise in the workout.

Tabata #68

Sprint

Grapevine

Air Squat

KB Thruster

Working at maximum capacity, exercise intensely for 20 seconds. Rest for 10 seconds. Repeat each exercise interval 8 times before moving to the next exercise in the workout.

Tabata #69

Air Squat
KB Clean & Press
Lunge
KB Swing

Workout Notes
**For KB Clean and Press, use one
or two kettlebells or dumbbells.**

Working at maximum capacity, exercise intensely for 20
seconds. Rest for 10 seconds. Repeat each exercise interval 8
times before moving to the next exercise in the workout.

Tabata #70

Grapevine (left)
High Knees
Grapevine (right)
Sprint

Workout Notes
Perform Sprint up a set of stairs,
up a hill, or on a flat surface.

Working at maximum capacity, exercise intensely for 20
seconds. Rest for 10 seconds. Repeat each exercise interval 8
times before moving to the next exercise in the workout.

Tabata #71

Lunge
Power Skip
KB Goblet Squat
Sprint

Working at maximum capacity, exercise intensely for 20 seconds. Rest for 10 seconds. Repeat each exercise interval 8 times before moving to the next exercise in the workout.

Tabata #72

Sprint
Sprint Backwards
Burpee
High Knees

Working at maximum capacity, exercise intensely for 20 seconds. Rest for 10 seconds. Repeat each exercise interval 8 times before moving to the next exercise in the workout.

Tabata #73

Burpee Long Jump
Power Skip
Karaoke Step
Sprint or Uphill Sprint

Working at maximum capacity, exercise intensely for 20 seconds. Rest for 10 seconds. Repeat each exercise interval 8 times before moving to the next exercise in the workout.

Tabata #74

KB Snatch
Plank-Up
Burpee Long Jump
KB Thruster

Workout Notes
For KB Thruster, use one or two kettlebells.

Working at maximum capacity, exercise intensely for 20 seconds. Rest for 10 seconds. Repeat each exercise interval 8 times before moving to the next exercise in the workout.

Tabata #75

KB Goblet Squat

Sprint

KB Push Press

Walking Lunge

Workout Notes
For Walking Lunge, hold the Push
Press weight for added difficulty.

Working at maximum capacity, exercise intensely for 20
seconds. Rest for 10 seconds. Repeat each exercise interval 8
times before moving to the next exercise in the workout.

Tabata #76

Bicycle Crunch
Long Jump
Spiderman Crawl
Bottom to Bottom Squat

Working at maximum capacity, exercise intensely for 20 seconds. Rest for 10 seconds. Repeat each exercise interval 8 times before moving to the next exercise in the workout.

Tabata #77

Bicycle Crunch

Grapevine

Burpee Long Jump

Sprint

Workout Notes
For Sprint, alternate sides each round.

Working at maximum capacity, exercise intensely for 20 seconds. Rest for 10 seconds. Repeat each exercise interval 8 times before moving to the next exercise in the workout.

Tabata #78

KB Snatch
Walking Lunge Step
Air Squat
Plyo-Push-Up

Workout Notes
For KB Snatch, alternate sides each round. For Walking Lunge Step, hold a weight for added difficulty.

Working at maximum capacity, exercise intensely for 20 seconds. Rest for 10 seconds. Repeat each exercise interval 8 times before moving to the next exercise in the workout.

Tabata #79

Sprint
Bent Over Row
KB Push Press
Step Up/Box Jump

Workout Notes
Perform Sprint up a hill or on a set of stairs, if available.
For KB Push Press, use two kettlebells. Step Up/Box Jump,
use a bench and alternate feet each step if stepping.

Working at maximum capacity, exercise intensely for 20
seconds. Rest for 10 seconds. Repeat each exercise interval 8
times before moving to the next exercise in the workout.

Tabata #80

Sprint
Burpee
Sit Up
KB Front Squat

Workout Notes
Perform Sprint up a hill or on a set of stairs, if available. For KB Front Squat, use two kettlebells.

Working at maximum capacity, exercise intensely for 20 seconds. Rest for 10 seconds. Repeat each exercise interval 8 times before moving to the next exercise in the workout.

Tabata #81

KB Thruster
Sprint
Long Jump
Bear Crawl

Workout Notes
For KB Thruster, use one kettlebell and alternate sides each round.

Working at maximum capacity, exercise intensely for 20 seconds. Rest for 10 seconds. Repeat each exercise interval 8 times before moving to the next exercise in the workout.

Tabata #82

Mountain Climber

Plank-Up

Sprint

Jumping Air Squat

Working at maximum capacity, exercise intensely for 20 seconds. Rest for 10 seconds. Repeat each exercise interval 8 times before moving to the next exercise in the workout.

Tabata #83

Spiderman Plank

Bottom To Bottom Squat

Long Jump

KB Clean

Workout Notes
For KB Clean, use a kettlebell or dumbbell and alternate sides each round.

Working at maximum capacity, exercise intensely for 20 seconds. Rest for 10 seconds. Repeat each exercise interval 8 times before moving to the next exercise in the workout.

Tabata #84

KB Clean & Thruster
High Knees
Long Jump
Mountain Climber

Workout Notes
For KB Clean and Thruster, re-clean the kettlebell from ground to shoulder on each repetition and alternate sides each round.

Working at maximum capacity, exercise intensely for 20 seconds. Rest for 10 seconds. Repeat each exercise interval 8 times before moving to the next exercise in the workout.

Tabata #85

KB Renegade Row
KB Swing
Mountain Climber
Sprint

Workout Notes
For KB Renegade Row,
alternate sides each repetition.

Working at maximum capacity, exercise intensely for 20 seconds. Rest for 10 seconds. Repeat each exercise interval 8 times before moving to the next exercise in the workout.

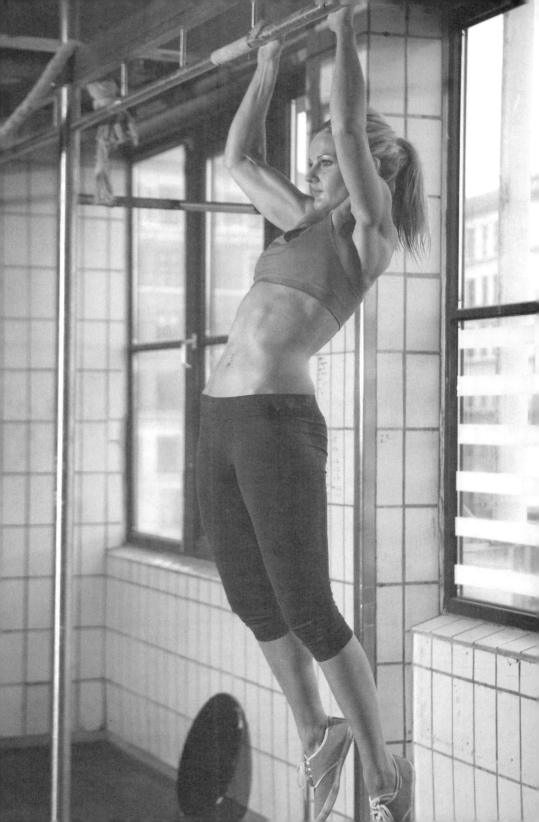

TABATAS
AT THE GYM

These tabatas incorporate free weights, machines, and other gym equipment found in traditional gyms. These workouts focus on your legs, arms and core, with a few full body workouts for a change of pace.

One problem that frequently occurs in a gym setting is that the equipment may be limited or already in use by someone else. In most cases, in the following workouts, if a machine is called for, it will typically be limited to one or two machines at the most, with the remainder of the movements able to be done with dumbbells, kettlebells, a bar, or even your own body weight.

Before beginning each workout, make sure to identify the equipment you need and to practice all four movements before getting started. If there is a time clock in the gym, you may use that to keep track of your intervals, though it will still be easier if you have an interval timer or a stopwatch.

Tabata #86

One-Leg Squat

Squat Jack

Barbell Back Squat

Squat Jack

Workout Notes
For One-Leg Squat, alternate sides each round.

Working at maximum capacity, exercise intensely for 20 seconds. Rest for 10 seconds. Repeat each exercise interval 8 times before moving to the next exercise in the workout.

Tabata #87

Leg Curl
Split Squat
Back Extension
Split Squat

Workout Notes
For Split Squat, alternate sides each round.

Working at maximum capacity, exercise intensely for 20 seconds. Rest for 10 seconds. Repeat each exercise interval 8 times before moving to the next exercise in the workout.

Tabata #88

Barbell Back Squat

Sumo Dead Lift

Leg Press with Toes Out

Reverse Lunge (with Weights)

Workout Notes
For Reverse Lunge with Weights, use two
dumbbells and alternate sides each step.

Working at maximum capacity, exercise intensely for 20
seconds. Rest for 10 seconds. Repeat each exercise interval 8
times before moving to the next exercise in the workout.

Tabata #89

Bench Step Up with Leg Raise

Dumbbell Sumo Squat

Back Extension

V-Up

Workout Notes
For Bench Step Up with Leg Raise, alternate sides each round. For Dumbbell Sumo Squat, hold a heavy kettlebell between your legs.

Working at maximum capacity, exercise intensely for 20 seconds. Rest for 10 seconds. Repeat each exercise interval 8 times before moving to the next exercise in the workout.

Tabata #90

Side Squat
Forward Lunge
One-Leg Squat
Jumping Squat

Workout Notes

For Side Squat, use a bar, kettlebell, dumbbell, or sandbag. For Forward Lunge, use two dumbbells. Perform One-Leg Squat with assistance if necessary. For Jumping Squat, hold a weight or medicine ball for added difficulty. Alternate sides each round.

Working at maximum capacity, exercise intensely for 20 seconds. Rest for 10 seconds. Repeat each exercise interval 8 times before moving to the next exercise in the workout.

Tabata #91

Pistol Squat
Kettlebell Swing
KB One-Leg Dead Lift
Squat Jack

Workout Notes
For Pistol Squat and KB One-Leg Dead Lift,
alternate sides each round.

Working at maximum capacity, exercise intensely for 20 seconds. Rest for 10 seconds. Repeat each exercise interval 8 times before moving to the next exercise in the workout.

Tabata #92

Lat Pull Down
Push-Up
Bent Over Row
Dumbbell Fly

Workout Notes
For Lat Pull Down, use a wide grip.

Working at maximum capacity, exercise intensely for 20 seconds. Rest for 10 seconds. Repeat each exercise interval 8 times before moving to the next exercise in the workout.

Tabata #93

Incline Press
Lat Pull Down
Dumbbell Fly
Dip

Workout Notes

For Incline Press, use dumbbells. For Lat Pull Down, use a narrow grip. For Dip, use a bench or Dip machine.

Working at maximum capacity, exercise intensely for 20 seconds. Rest for 10 seconds. Repeat each exercise interval 8 times before moving to the next exercise in the workout.

Tabata #94

Lat Pull Down
Seated Bicep Curl
Pull-Up/Lat Pull-Down
Hang Clean

Workout Notes

For Lat Pull Down, use a wide grip. For Hang Clean, use a dumbbell or barbell.

Working at maximum capacity, exercise intensely for 20 seconds. Rest for 10 seconds. Repeat each exercise interval 8 times before moving to the next exercise in the workout.

Tabata #95

Skull Crusher

Standing Bicep Curl

Diamond Push-Up

Pull-Up/Lat Pull-Down

Workout Notes
For Skull Crusher, lay on your back on a bench and extend your hands over your head.

Working at maximum capacity, exercise intensely for 20 seconds. Rest for 10 seconds. Repeat each exercise interval 8 times before moving to the next exercise in the workout.

Tabata #96

Overhead Press

Roman Chair Knee Raise

Lateral Raise

Rear Deltoid Fly

Workout Notes
For Overhead Press, use a barbell or two dumbbells.
For Lateral Raise, use dumbbells.

Working at maximum capacity, exercise intensely for 20 seconds. Rest for 10 seconds. Repeat each exercise interval 8 times before moving to the next exercise in the workout.

Tabata #97

Reverse Sit-Up

Roman Chair Knee/Leg Raise

Weighted Sit Up

Spiderman Plank

Workout Notes
Perform Weighted Sit Up while holding a weight behind your head.

Working at maximum capacity, exercise intensely for 20 seconds. Rest for 10 seconds. Repeat each exercise interval 8 times before moving to the next exercise in the workout.

Tabata #98

Triceps Dips (on Bench or Box)

KB Thruster

KB Front Squat

Standing Bicep Curl

Workout Notes

**For KB Thruster and KB Front Squat, use a barbell.
For Standing Bicep Curl, use a barbell or dumbbells.**

Working at maximum capacity, exercise intensely for 20
seconds. Rest for 10 seconds. Repeat each exercise interval 8
times before moving to the next exercise in the workout.

Tabata #99

Dumbbell Bench Press
Bent Over Row
Hand Release Push-Up
Hang Clean

Workout Notes

For Hang Clean, use dumbbells or a barbell. If using dumbbells, use two and do both arms each round.

Working at maximum capacity, exercise intensely for 20 seconds. Rest for 10 seconds. Repeat each exercise interval 8 times before moving to the next exercise in the workout.

Tabata #100

Bent Over Row
Lateral Jump
Shoulder Press
Roman Chair Knee/Leg Raise

Workout Notes
For Bent Over Row and Shoulder Press, use a barbell or two dumbbells. For Lateral Jump, jump over a dumbbell, side to side.

Working at maximum capacity, exercise intensely for 20 seconds. Rest for 10 seconds. Repeat each exercise interval 8 times before moving to the next exercise in the workout.

Tabata #101

Seated Bicep Curl

Walking Lunge

Kettlebell Swing

Decline Push-Up

Workout Notes
Perform Walking Lunge while holding a plate over your head.

Working at maximum capacity, exercise intensely for 20 seconds. Rest for 10 seconds. Repeat each exercise interval 8 times before moving to the next exercise in the workout.

Tabata #102

Shoulder Press

Roman Chair Knee/Leg Raise

Pull-Up/Lat Pull-Down

Dumbbell Sumo Squat

Workout Notes
For Shoulder Press, use a barbell or two dumbbells.
Perform Dumbbell Sumo Squat with one heavy weight.

Working at maximum capacity, exercise intensely for 20 seconds. Rest for 10 seconds. Repeat each exercise interval 8 times before moving to the next exercise in the workout.

Tabata #103

KB Russian Twist

Bench Step Up with Knee Raise

Weighted Sit Up

Sumo Dead Lift

Workout Notes
For Bench Step Up with Knee Raise,
alternate sides each round.

Working at maximum capacity, exercise intensely for 20 seconds. Rest for 10 seconds. Repeat each exercise interval 8 times before moving to the next exercise in the workout.

Tabata #104

Dumbbell Hang Clean
Shoulder Press
KB Front Squat
KB Swing

Workout Notes

For Dumbbell Hang Clean and KB Front Squat, use two kettlebells and hold the bells in rack during any rest periods. For Shoulder Press, use two kettlebells or dumbbells and hold the bells in rack during any rest periods.

Working at maximum capacity, exercise intensely for 20 seconds. Rest for 10 seconds. Repeat each exercise interval 8 times before moving to the next exercise in the workout.

Tabata #105

Pistol Squat
Shoulder Press
KB Front Squat
Barbell Hang Clean

Workout Notes
For Pistol Squat, alternate sides each round. For Shoulder Press, use two kettlebells or dumbbells. For KB Front Squat, use two kettlebells.

Working at maximum capacity, exercise intensely for 20 seconds. Rest for 10 seconds. Repeat each exercise interval 8 times before moving to the next exercise in the workout.

Tabata #106

Skull Crusher
Leg Press
Seated Bicep Curl
KB Dead Lift

Working at maximum capacity, exercise intensely for 20 seconds. Rest for 10 seconds. Repeat each exercise interval 8 times before moving to the next exercise in the workout.

Tabata #107

Bent Over Row
Incline Press
Dip
Squat Jack

Working at maximum capacity, exercise intensely for 20 seconds. Rest for 10 seconds. Repeat each exercise interval 8 times before moving to the next exercise in the workout.

Tabata #108

KB One-Leg Dead Lift
One-Leg Squat
KB Renegade Row
KB Thruster

Workout Notes

For KB Renegade Row, alternate sides each round. For KB Thruster, alternate sides each round or use two kettlebells.

Working at maximum capacity, exercise intensely for 20 seconds. Rest for 10 seconds. Repeat each exercise interval 8 times before moving to the next exercise in the workout.

Tabata #109

Barbell Back Squat

Step Up (with Knee Raise)

Dumbbell Sumo Squat

Sumo Dead Lift

Workout Notes
For Step Up with Knee Raise, alternate sides each round.

Working at maximum capacity, exercise intensely for 20 seconds. Rest for 10 seconds. Repeat each exercise interval 8 times before moving to the next exercise in the workout.

Tabata #110

Overhead Walking Lunge

Back Extension

Weighted Sit Up

Spiderman Plank

Workout Notes
For Overhead Walking Lunge, hold one
45-pound plate overhead. For Spiderman
Plank, alternate sides each repetition.

Working at maximum capacity, exercise intensely for 20
seconds. Rest for 10 seconds. Repeat each exercise interval 8
times before moving to the next exercise in the workout.

ADDING INTENSITY TO YOUR WORKOUTS

Below are a few easy ways to make your workouts more challenging. Try them out and find what works best for you. The key to continuing progress is to keep challenging yourself; don't be afraid to mix it up!

1. Do more work at a faster pace during the work period.

2. Change up your weights: Go lighter and work more intensely or increase your weights for a harder workout. This will reduce your rep count, but this is okay if you are working intensely with good form.

3. Do a more difficult variation of the movement. There are many variations of each movement available for when changing weight isn't enough. For example, there are hundreds of variations of push-ups; choose one that is more difficult and substitute it for the standard push-up. If the Handstand Hold is too easy, find out how to perform Handstand Push-Ups.

4. Increase core tension. In addition to making you keep better form and protecting your body more, using maximum core tension for every movement will drastically increase the intensity of your workout.

5. Stay active during recovery time. This could be anything from fast walking, to slow jumping jacks, to holding the plank position. If you are at the point where a movement is too easy, but you are not ready to increase the weight or try a more difficult variation, this is a great way to add intensity to your tabata workout.

TABATA TRACKER

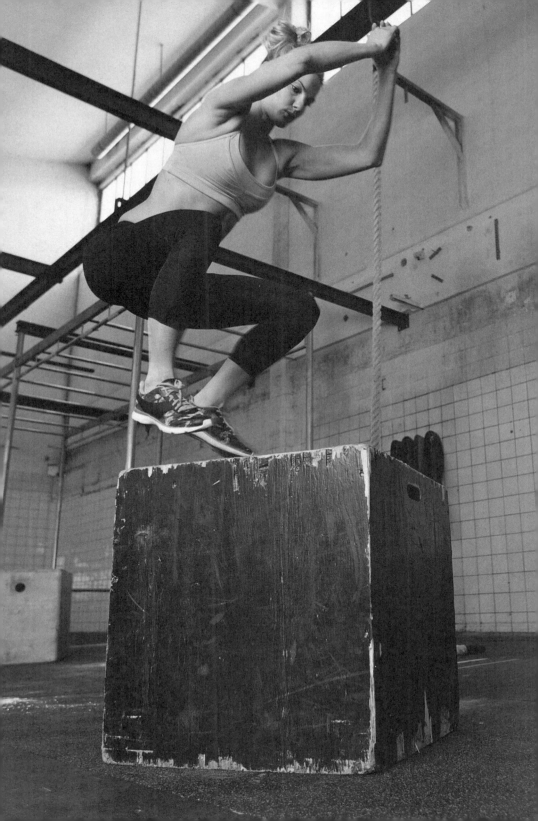

EXAMPLE

Tabata Tracker   Date: ___5/1___   Tabata Workout # ____1____

Exercise 1: Squat Thrust	Exercise 2: Air Squat	Exercise 3: Sit Up	Exercise 4: Push-Up
Total Reps: 7	Total Reps: 15	Total Reps: 10	Total Reps: 5
Weight: none	Weight: none	Weight: 10 pounds (kettlebell)	Weight: none

One of the best tips I can give for keeping track of your fitness level and your progress is to record your workouts. I would also encourage you to record your diet (not just the healthy things you eat, but everything you drink, eat for meals, and for snacks).

Please use this book to record your workouts, including your maximum reps and maximum weight used. On the following pages, we have provided space for you to record your reps and weights for each workout. These should serve as markers, so that the next time you return to a workout (in 4 to 6 weeks, for example), you can determine whether you've improved; and if so, by how much. Even having this small indication of personal progress can be incredibly empowering, and you'll find your confidence increasing in track with your own fitness level.

Remember, progress is not always linear; if you don't improve every day, stick with it! Getting fitter and stronger takes time! If you eat well, work out regularly, and stay focused on your goals, you will get great results!

Tabata Tracker   Date: _____   Tabata Workout # _____

Exercise 1:	Exercise 2:	Exercise 3:	Exercise 4:
Total Reps:	Total Reps:	Total Reps:	Total Reps:
Weight:	Weight:	Weight:	Weight:

Tabata Tracker   Date: _____   Tabata Workout # _____

Exercise 1:	Exercise 2:	Exercise 3:	Exercise 4:
Total Reps:	Total Reps:	Total Reps:	Total Reps:
Weight:	Weight:	Weight:	Weight:

Tabata Tracker   Date: _____   Tabata Workout # _____

Exercise 1:	Exercise 2:	Exercise 3:	Exercise 4:
Total Reps:	Total Reps:	Total Reps:	Total Reps:
Weight:	Weight:	Weight:	Weight:

Tabata Tracker   Date: _____   Tabata Workout # _____

Exercise 1:	Exercise 2:	Exercise 3:	Exercise 4:
Total Reps:	Total Reps:	Total Reps:	Total Reps:
Weight:	Weight:	Weight:	Weight:

Tabata Tracker   Date: _____   Tabata Workout # _____

Exercise 1:	Exercise 2:	Exercise 3:	Exercise 4:
Total Reps:	Total Reps:	Total Reps:	Total Reps:
Weight:	Weight:	Weight:	Weight:

Tabata Tracker   Date: _____   Tabata Workout # _____

Exercise 1:	Exercise 2:	Exercise 3:	Exercise 4:
Total Reps:	Total Reps:	Total Reps:	Total Reps:
Weight:	Weight:	Weight:	Weight:

Tabata Tracker   Date: _____   Tabata Workout # _____

Exercise 1:	Exercise 2:	Exercise 3:	Exercise 4:
Total Reps:	Total Reps:	Total Reps:	Total Reps:
Weight:	Weight:	Weight:	Weight:

Tabata Tracker   Date: _____   Tabata Workout # _____

Exercise 1:	Exercise 2:	Exercise 3:	Exercise 4:
Total Reps:	Total Reps:	Total Reps:	Total Reps:
Weight:	Weight:	Weight:	Weight:

Tabata Tracker   Date: _____   Tabata Workout # _____

Exercise 1:	Exercise 2:	Exercise 3:	Exercise 4:
Total Reps:	Total Reps:	Total Reps:	Total Reps:
Weight:	Weight:	Weight:	Weight:

Tabata Tracker   Date: _____   Tabata Workout # _____

Exercise 1:	Exercise 2:	Exercise 3:	Exercise 4:
Total Reps:	Total Reps:	Total Reps:	Total Reps:
Weight:	Weight:	Weight:	Weight:

Tabata Tracker   Date: _____   Tabata Workout # _____

Exercise 1:	Exercise 2:	Exercise 3:	Exercise 4:
Total Reps:	Total Reps:	Total Reps:	Total Reps:
Weight:	Weight:	Weight:	Weight:

Tabata Tracker   Date: _____   Tabata Workout # _____

Exercise 1:	Exercise 2:	Exercise 3:	Exercise 4:
Total Reps:	Total Reps:	Total Reps:	Total Reps:
Weight:	Weight:	Weight:	Weight:

Tabata Tracker   Date: _____   Tabata Workout # _____

Exercise 1:	Exercise 2:	Exercise 3:	Exercise 4:
Total Reps:	Total Reps:	Total Reps:	Total Reps:
Weight:	Weight:	Weight:	Weight:

Tabata Tracker   Date: _____   Tabata Workout # _____

Exercise 1:	Exercise 2:	Exercise 3:	Exercise 4:
Total Reps:	Total Reps:	Total Reps:	Total Reps:
Weight:	Weight:	Weight:	Weight:

Tabata Tracker   Date: _____   Tabata Workout # _____

Exercise 1:	Exercise 2:	Exercise 3:	Exercise 4:
Total Reps:	Total Reps:	Total Reps:	Total Reps:
Weight:	Weight:	Weight:	Weight:

Tabata Tracker   Date: _____   Tabata Workout # _____

Exercise 1:	Exercise 2:	Exercise 3:	Exercise 4:
Total Reps:	Total Reps:	Total Reps:	Total Reps:
Weight:	Weight:	Weight:	Weight:

Tabata Tracker Date: _____ Tabata Workout # _____

Exercise 1:	Exercise 2:	Exercise 3:	Exercise 4:
Total Reps:	Total Reps:	Total Reps:	Total Reps:
Weight:	Weight:	Weight:	Weight:

Tabata Tracker Date: _____ Tabata Workout # _____

Exercise 1:	Exercise 2:	Exercise 3:	Exercise 4:
Total Reps:	Total Reps:	Total Reps:	Total Reps:
Weight:	Weight:	Weight:	Weight:

Tabata Tracker Date: _____ Tabata Workout # _____

Exercise 1:	Exercise 2:	Exercise 3:	Exercise 4:
Total Reps:	Total Reps:	Total Reps:	Total Reps:
Weight:	Weight:	Weight:	Weight:

Tabata Tracker Date: _____ Tabata Workout # _____

Exercise 1:	Exercise 2:	Exercise 3:	Exercise 4:
Total Reps:	Total Reps:	Total Reps:	Total Reps:
Weight:	Weight:	Weight:	Weight:

Tabata Tracker Date: _____   Tabata Workout # _____

Exercise 1:	Exercise 2:	Exercise 3:	Exercise 4:
Total Reps:	Total Reps:	Total Reps:	Total Reps:
Weight:	Weight:	Weight:	Weight:

Tabata Tracker Date: _____   Tabata Workout # _____

Exercise 1:	Exercise 2:	Exercise 3:	Exercise 4:
Total Reps:	Total Reps:	Total Reps:	Total Reps:
Weight:	Weight:	Weight:	Weight:

Tabata Tracker Date: _____   Tabata Workout # _____

Exercise 1:	Exercise 2:	Exercise 3:	Exercise 4:
Total Reps:	Total Reps:	Total Reps:	Total Reps:
Weight:	Weight:	Weight:	Weight:

Tabata Tracker Date: _____   Tabata Workout # _____

Exercise 1:	Exercise 2:	Exercise 3:	Exercise 4:
Total Reps:	Total Reps:	Total Reps:	Total Reps:
Weight:	Weight:	Weight:	Weight:

TABATA WORKOUT HANDBOOK

Tabata Tracker   Date: _____   Tabata Workout # _____

Exercise 1:	Exercise 2:	Exercise 3:	Exercise 4:
Total Reps:	Total Reps:	Total Reps:	Total Reps:
Weight:	Weight:	Weight:	Weight:

Tabata Tracker   Date: _____   Tabata Workout # _____

Exercise 1:	Exercise 2:	Exercise 3:	Exercise 4:
Total Reps:	Total Reps:	Total Reps:	Total Reps:
Weight:	Weight:	Weight:	Weight:

Tabata Tracker   Date: _____   Tabata Workout # _____

Exercise 1:	Exercise 2:	Exercise 3:	Exercise 4:
Total Reps:	Total Reps:	Total Reps:	Total Reps:
Weight:	Weight:	Weight:	Weight:

Tabata Tracker   Date: _____   Tabata Workout # _____

Exercise 1:	Exercise 2:	Exercise 3:	Exercise 4:
Total Reps:	Total Reps:	Total Reps:	Total Reps:
Weight:	Weight:	Weight:	Weight:

Tabata Tracker Date: _____ Tabata Workout # _____

Exercise 1:	Exercise 2:	Exercise 3:	Exercise 4:
Total Reps:	Total Reps:	Total Reps:	Total Reps:
Weight:	Weight:	Weight:	Weight:

Tabata Tracker Date: _____ Tabata Workout # _____

Exercise 1:	Exercise 2:	Exercise 3:	Exercise 4:
Total Reps:	Total Reps:	Total Reps:	Total Reps:
Weight:	Weight:	Weight:	Weight:

Tabata Tracker Date: _____ Tabata Workout # _____

Exercise 1:	Exercise 2:	Exercise 3:	Exercise 4:
Total Reps:	Total Reps:	Total Reps:	Total Reps:
Weight:	Weight:	Weight:	Weight:

Tabata Tracker Date: _____ Tabata Workout # _____

Exercise 1:	Exercise 2:	Exercise 3:	Exercise 4:
Total Reps:	Total Reps:	Total Reps:	Total Reps:
Weight:	Weight:	Weight:	Weight:

TABATA WORKOUT HANDBOOK

Tabata Tracker Date: _____ Tabata Workout # _____

Exercise 1:	Exercise 2:	Exercise 3:	Exercise 4:
Total Reps:	Total Reps:	Total Reps:	Total Reps:
Weight:	Weight:	Weight:	Weight:

Tabata Tracker Date: _____ Tabata Workout # _____

Exercise 1:	Exercise 2:	Exercise 3:	Exercise 4:
Total Reps:	Total Reps:	Total Reps:	Total Reps:
Weight:	Weight:	Weight:	Weight:

Tabata Tracker Date: _____ Tabata Workout # _____

Exercise 1:	Exercise 2:	Exercise 3:	Exercise 4:
Total Reps:	Total Reps:	Total Reps:	Total Reps:
Weight:	Weight:	Weight:	Weight:

Tabata Tracker Date: _____ Tabata Workout # _____

Exercise 1:	Exercise 2:	Exercise 3:	Exercise 4:
Total Reps:	Total Reps:	Total Reps:	Total Reps:
Weight:	Weight:	Weight:	Weight:

Tabata Tracker   Date: _____   Tabata Workout # _____

Exercise 1:	Exercise 2:	Exercise 3:	Exercise 4:
Total Reps:	Total Reps:	Total Reps:	Total Reps:
Weight:	Weight:	Weight:	Weight:

Tabata Tracker   Date: _____   Tabata Workout # _____

Exercise 1:	Exercise 2:	Exercise 3:	Exercise 4:
Total Reps:	Total Reps:	Total Reps:	Total Reps:
Weight:	Weight:	Weight:	Weight:

Tabata Tracker   Date: _____   Tabata Workout # _____

Exercise 1:	Exercise 2:	Exercise 3:	Exercise 4:
Total Reps:	Total Reps:	Total Reps:	Total Reps:
Weight:	Weight:	Weight:	Weight:

Tabata Tracker   Date: _____   Tabata Workout # _____

Exercise 1:	Exercise 2:	Exercise 3:	Exercise 4:
Total Reps:	Total Reps:	Total Reps:	Total Reps:
Weight:	Weight:	Weight:	Weight:

TABATA WORKOUT HANDBOOK

Tabata Tracker   Date: _____   Tabata Workout # _____

Exercise 1:	Exercise 2:	Exercise 3:	Exercise 4:
Total Reps:	Total Reps:	Total Reps:	Total Reps:
Weight:	Weight:	Weight:	Weight:

Tabata Tracker   Date: _____   Tabata Workout # _____

Exercise 1:	Exercise 2:	Exercise 3:	Exercise 4:
Total Reps:	Total Reps:	Total Reps:	Total Reps:
Weight:	Weight:	Weight:	Weight:

Tabata Tracker   Date: _____   Tabata Workout # _____

Exercise 1:	Exercise 2:	Exercise 3:	Exercise 4:
Total Reps:	Total Reps:	Total Reps:	Total Reps:
Weight:	Weight:	Weight:	Weight:

Tabata Tracker   Date: _____   Tabata Workout # _____

Exercise 1:	Exercise 2:	Exercise 3:	Exercise 4:
Total Reps:	Total Reps:	Total Reps:	Total Reps:
Weight:	Weight:	Weight:	Weight:

Tabata Tracker   Date: _____   Tabata Workout # _____

Exercise 1:	Exercise 2:	Exercise 3:	Exercise 4:
Total Reps:	Total Reps:	Total Reps:	Total Reps:
Weight:	Weight:	Weight:	Weight:

Tabata Tracker   Date: _____   Tabata Workout # _____

Exercise 1:	Exercise 2:	Exercise 3:	Exercise 4:
Total Reps:	Total Reps:	Total Reps:	Total Reps:
Weight:	Weight:	Weight:	Weight:

Tabata Tracker   Date: _____   Tabata Workout # _____

Exercise 1:	Exercise 2:	Exercise 3:	Exercise 4:
Total Reps:	Total Reps:	Total Reps:	Total Reps:
Weight:	Weight:	Weight:	Weight:

Tabata Tracker   Date: _____   Tabata Workout # _____

Exercise 1:	Exercise 2:	Exercise 3:	Exercise 4:
Total Reps:	Total Reps:	Total Reps:	Total Reps:
Weight:	Weight:	Weight:	Weight:

Tabata Tracker   Date: _____   Tabata Workout # _____

Exercise 1:	Exercise 2:	Exercise 3:	Exercise 4:
Total Reps:	Total Reps:	Total Reps:	Total Reps:
Weight:	Weight:	Weight:	Weight:

Tabata Tracker   Date: _____   Tabata Workout # _____

Exercise 1:	Exercise 2:	Exercise 3:	Exercise 4:
Total Reps:	Total Reps:	Total Reps:	Total Reps:
Weight:	Weight:	Weight:	Weight:

Tabata Tracker   Date: _____   Tabata Workout # _____

Exercise 1:	Exercise 2:	Exercise 3:	Exercise 4:
Total Reps:	Total Reps:	Total Reps:	Total Reps:
Weight:	Weight:	Weight:	Weight:

Tabata Tracker   Date: _____   Tabata Workout # _____

Exercise 1:	Exercise 2:	Exercise 3:	Exercise 4:
Total Reps:	Total Reps:	Total Reps:	Total Reps:
Weight:	Weight:	Weight:	Weight:

Tabata Tracker   Date: _____   Tabata Workout # _____

Exercise 1:	Exercise 2:	Exercise 3:	Exercise 4:
Total Reps:	Total Reps:	Total Reps:	Total Reps:
Weight:	Weight:	Weight:	Weight:

Tabata Tracker   Date: _____   Tabata Workout # _____

Exercise 1:	Exercise 2:	Exercise 3:	Exercise 4:
Total Reps:	Total Reps:	Total Reps:	Total Reps:
Weight:	Weight:	Weight:	Weight:

Tabata Tracker   Date: _____   Tabata Workout # _____

Exercise 1:	Exercise 2:	Exercise 3:	Exercise 4:
Total Reps:	Total Reps:	Total Reps:	Total Reps:
Weight:	Weight:	Weight:	Weight:

Tabata Tracker   Date: _____   Tabata Workout # _____

Exercise 1:	Exercise 2:	Exercise 3:	Exercise 4:
Total Reps:	Total Reps:	Total Reps:	Total Reps:
Weight:	Weight:	Weight:	Weight:

TABATA WORKOUT HANDBOOK

Tabata Tracker   Date: _____   Tabata Workout # _____

Exercise 1:	Exercise 2:	Exercise 3:	Exercise 4:
Total Reps:	Total Reps:	Total Reps:	Total Reps:
Weight:	Weight:	Weight:	Weight:

Tabata Tracker   Date: _____   Tabata Workout # _____

Exercise 1:	Exercise 2:	Exercise 3:	Exercise 4:
Total Reps:	Total Reps:	Total Reps:	Total Reps:
Weight:	Weight:	Weight:	Weight:

Tabata Tracker   Date: _____   Tabata Workout # _____

Exercise 1:	Exercise 2:	Exercise 3:	Exercise 4:
Total Reps:	Total Reps:	Total Reps:	Total Reps:
Weight:	Weight:	Weight:	Weight:

Tabata Tracker   Date: _____   Tabata Workout # _____

Exercise 1:	Exercise 2:	Exercise 3:	Exercise 4:
Total Reps:	Total Reps:	Total Reps:	Total Reps:
Weight:	Weight:	Weight:	Weight:

Tabata Tracker   Date: _____   Tabata Workout # _____

Exercise 1:	Exercise 2:	Exercise 3:	Exercise 4:
Total Reps:	Total Reps:	Total Reps:	Total Reps:
Weight:	Weight:	Weight:	Weight:

Tabata Tracker   Date: _____   Tabata Workout # _____

Exercise 1:	Exercise 2:	Exercise 3:	Exercise 4:
Total Reps:	Total Reps:	Total Reps:	Total Reps:
Weight:	Weight:	Weight:	Weight:

Tabata Tracker   Date: _____   Tabata Workout # _____

Exercise 1:	Exercise 2:	Exercise 3:	Exercise 4:
Total Reps:	Total Reps:	Total Reps:	Total Reps:
Weight:	Weight:	Weight:	Weight:

Tabata Tracker   Date: _____   Tabata Workout # _____

Exercise 1:	Exercise 2:	Exercise 3:	Exercise 4:
Total Reps:	Total Reps:	Total Reps:	Total Reps:
Weight:	Weight:	Weight:	Weight:

TABATA WORKOUT HANDBOOK

Tabata Tracker   Date: _____   Tabata Workout # _____

Exercise 1:	Exercise 2:	Exercise 3:	Exercise 4:
Total Reps:	Total Reps:	Total Reps:	Total Reps:
Weight:	Weight:	Weight:	Weight:

Tabata Tracker   Date: _____   Tabata Workout # _____

Exercise 1:	Exercise 2:	Exercise 3:	Exercise 4:
Total Reps:	Total Reps:	Total Reps:	Total Reps:
Weight:	Weight:	Weight:	Weight:

Tabata Tracker   Date: _____   Tabata Workout # _____

Exercise 1:	Exercise 2:	Exercise 3:	Exercise 4:
Total Reps:	Total Reps:	Total Reps:	Total Reps:
Weight:	Weight:	Weight:	Weight:

Tabata Tracker   Date: _____   Tabata Workout # _____

Exercise 1:	Exercise 2:	Exercise 3:	Exercise 4:
Total Reps:	Total Reps:	Total Reps:	Total Reps:
Weight:	Weight:	Weight:	Weight:

Tabata Tracker Date: _____ Tabata Workout # _____

Exercise 1:	Exercise 2:	Exercise 3:	Exercise 4:
Total Reps:	Total Reps:	Total Reps:	Total Reps:
Weight:	Weight:	Weight:	Weight:

Tabata Tracker Date: _____ Tabata Workout # _____

Exercise 1:	Exercise 2:	Exercise 3:	Exercise 4:
Total Reps:	Total Reps:	Total Reps:	Total Reps:
Weight:	Weight:	Weight:	Weight:

Tabata Tracker Date: _____ Tabata Workout # _____

Exercise 1:	Exercise 2:	Exercise 3:	Exercise 4:
Total Reps:	Total Reps:	Total Reps:	Total Reps:
Weight:	Weight:	Weight:	Weight:

Tabata Tracker Date: _____ Tabata Workout # _____

Exercise 1:	Exercise 2:	Exercise 3:	Exercise 4:
Total Reps:	Total Reps:	Total Reps:	Total Reps:
Weight:	Weight:	Weight:	Weight:

TABATA WORKOUT HANDBOOK

Tabata Tracker Date: _____ Tabata Workout # _____

Exercise 1:	Exercise 2:	Exercise 3:	Exercise 4:
Total Reps:	Total Reps:	Total Reps:	Total Reps:
Weight:	Weight:	Weight:	Weight:

Tabata Tracker Date: _____ Tabata Workout # _____

Exercise 1:	Exercise 2:	Exercise 3:	Exercise 4:
Total Reps:	Total Reps:	Total Reps:	Total Reps:
Weight:	Weight:	Weight:	Weight:

Tabata Tracker Date: _____ Tabata Workout # _____

Exercise 1:	Exercise 2:	Exercise 3:	Exercise 4:
Total Reps:	Total Reps:	Total Reps:	Total Reps:
Weight:	Weight:	Weight:	Weight:

Tabata Tracker Date: _____ Tabata Workout # _____

Exercise 1:	Exercise 2:	Exercise 3:	Exercise 4:
Total Reps:	Total Reps:	Total Reps:	Total Reps:
Weight:	Weight:	Weight:	Weight:

Tabata Tracker   Date: _____   Tabata Workout # _____

Exercise 1:	Exercise 2:	Exercise 3:	Exercise 4:
Total Reps:	Total Reps:	Total Reps:	Total Reps:
Weight:	Weight:	Weight:	Weight:

Tabata Tracker   Date: _____   Tabata Workout # _____

Exercise 1:	Exercise 2:	Exercise 3:	Exercise 4:
Total Reps:	Total Reps:	Total Reps:	Total Reps:
Weight:	Weight:	Weight:	Weight:

Tabata Tracker   Date: _____   Tabata Workout # _____

Exercise 1:	Exercise 2:	Exercise 3:	Exercise 4:
Total Reps:	Total Reps:	Total Reps:	Total Reps:
Weight:	Weight:	Weight:	Weight:

Tabata Tracker   Date: _____   Tabata Workout # _____

Exercise 1:	Exercise 2:	Exercise 3:	Exercise 4:
Total Reps:	Total Reps:	Total Reps:	Total Reps:
Weight:	Weight:	Weight:	Weight:

Tabata Tracker Date: _____ Tabata Workout # _____

Exercise 1:	Exercise 2:	Exercise 3:	Exercise 4:
Total Reps:	Total Reps:	Total Reps:	Total Reps:
Weight:	Weight:	Weight:	Weight:

Tabata Tracker Date: _____ Tabata Workout # _____

Exercise 1:	Exercise 2:	Exercise 3:	Exercise 4:
Total Reps:	Total Reps:	Total Reps:	Total Reps:
Weight:	Weight:	Weight:	Weight:

Tabata Tracker Date: _____ Tabata Workout # _____

Exercise 1:	Exercise 2:	Exercise 3:	Exercise 4:
Total Reps:	Total Reps:	Total Reps:	Total Reps:
Weight:	Weight:	Weight:	Weight:

Tabata Tracker Date: _____ Tabata Workout # _____

Exercise 1:	Exercise 2:	Exercise 3:	Exercise 4:
Total Reps:	Total Reps:	Total Reps:	Total Reps:
Weight:	Weight:	Weight:	Weight:

Tabata Tracker Date: _____ Tabata Workout # _____

Exercise 1:	Exercise 2:	Exercise 3:	Exercise 4:
Total Reps:	Total Reps:	Total Reps:	Total Reps:
Weight:	Weight:	Weight:	Weight:

Tabata Tracker Date: _____ Tabata Workout # _____

Exercise 1:	Exercise 2:	Exercise 3:	Exercise 4:
Total Reps:	Total Reps:	Total Reps:	Total Reps:
Weight:	Weight:	Weight:	Weight:

Tabata Tracker Date: _____ Tabata Workout # _____

Exercise 1:	Exercise 2:	Exercise 3:	Exercise 4:
Total Reps:	Total Reps:	Total Reps:	Total Reps:
Weight:	Weight:	Weight:	Weight:

Tabata Tracker Date: _____ Tabata Workout # _____

Exercise 1:	Exercise 2:	Exercise 3:	Exercise 4:
Total Reps:	Total Reps:	Total Reps:	Total Reps:
Weight:	Weight:	Weight:	Weight:

Tabata Tracker Date: _____ Tabata Workout # _____

Exercise 1:	Exercise 2:	Exercise 3:	Exercise 4:
Total Reps:	Total Reps:	Total Reps:	Total Reps:
Weight:	Weight:	Weight:	Weight:

Tabata Tracker Date: _____ Tabata Workout # _____

Exercise 1:	Exercise 2:	Exercise 3:	Exercise 4:
Total Reps:	Total Reps:	Total Reps:	Total Reps:
Weight:	Weight:	Weight:	Weight:

Tabata Tracker Date: _____ Tabata Workout # _____

Exercise 1:	Exercise 2:	Exercise 3:	Exercise 4:
Total Reps:	Total Reps:	Total Reps:	Total Reps:
Weight:	Weight:	Weight:	Weight:

Tabata Tracker Date: _____ Tabata Workout # _____

Exercise 1:	Exercise 2:	Exercise 3:	Exercise 4:
Total Reps:	Total Reps:	Total Reps:	Total Reps:
Weight:	Weight:	Weight:	Weight:

Tabata Tracker   Date: _____   Tabata Workout # _____

Exercise 1:	Exercise 2:	Exercise 3:	Exercise 4:
Total Reps:	Total Reps:	Total Reps:	Total Reps:
Weight:	Weight:	Weight:	Weight:

Tabata Tracker   Date: _____   Tabata Workout # _____

Exercise 1:	Exercise 2:	Exercise 3:	Exercise 4:
Total Reps:	Total Reps:	Total Reps:	Total Reps:
Weight:	Weight:	Weight:	Weight:

Tabata Tracker   Date: _____   Tabata Workout # _____

Exercise 1:	Exercise 2:	Exercise 3:	Exercise 4:
Total Reps:	Total Reps:	Total Reps:	Total Reps:
Weight:	Weight:	Weight:	Weight:

Tabata Tracker   Date: _____   Tabata Workout # _____

Exercise 1:	Exercise 2:	Exercise 3:	Exercise 4:
Total Reps:	Total Reps:	Total Reps:	Total Reps:
Weight:	Weight:	Weight:	Weight:

Tabata Tracker Date: _____ Tabata Workout # _____

Exercise 1:	Exercise 2:	Exercise 3:	Exercise 4:
Total Reps:	Total Reps:	Total Reps:	Total Reps:
Weight:	Weight:	Weight:	Weight:

Tabata Tracker Date: _____ Tabata Workout # _____

Exercise 1:	Exercise 2:	Exercise 3:	Exercise 4:
Total Reps:	Total Reps:	Total Reps:	Total Reps:
Weight:	Weight:	Weight:	Weight:

Tabata Tracker Date: _____ Tabata Workout # _____

Exercise 1:	Exercise 2:	Exercise 3:	Exercise 4:
Total Reps:	Total Reps:	Total Reps:	Total Reps:
Weight:	Weight:	Weight:	Weight:

Tabata Tracker Date: _____ Tabata Workout # _____

Exercise 1:	Exercise 2:	Exercise 3:	Exercise 4:
Total Reps:	Total Reps:	Total Reps:	Total Reps:
Weight:	Weight:	Weight:	Weight:

Tabata Tracker   Date: _____   Tabata Workout # _____

Exercise 1:	Exercise 2:	Exercise 3:	Exercise 4:
Total Reps:	Total Reps:	Total Reps:	Total Reps:
Weight:	Weight:	Weight:	Weight:

Tabata Tracker   Date: _____   Tabata Workout # _____

Exercise 1:	Exercise 2:	Exercise 3:	Exercise 4:
Total Reps:	Total Reps:	Total Reps:	Total Reps:
Weight:	Weight:	Weight:	Weight:

Tabata Tracker   Date: _____   Tabata Workout # _____

Exercise 1:	Exercise 2:	Exercise 3:	Exercise 4:
Total Reps:	Total Reps:	Total Reps:	Total Reps:
Weight:	Weight:	Weight:	Weight:

Tabata Tracker   Date: _____   Tabata Workout # _____

Exercise 1:	Exercise 2:	Exercise 3:	Exercise 4:
Total Reps:	Total Reps:	Total Reps:	Total Reps:
Weight:	Weight:	Weight:	Weight:

Tabata Tracker Date: _____ Tabata Workout # _____

Exercise 1:	Exercise 2:	Exercise 3:	Exercise 4:
Total Reps:	Total Reps:	Total Reps:	Total Reps:
Weight:	Weight:	Weight:	Weight:

Tabata Tracker Date: _____ Tabata Workout # _____

Exercise 1:	Exercise 2:	Exercise 3:	Exercise 4:
Total Reps:	Total Reps:	Total Reps:	Total Reps:
Weight:	Weight:	Weight:	Weight:

Tabata Tracker Date: _____ Tabata Workout # _____

Exercise 1:	Exercise 2:	Exercise 3:	Exercise 4:
Total Reps:	Total Reps:	Total Reps:	Total Reps:
Weight:	Weight:	Weight:	Weight:

Tabata Tracker Date: _____ Tabata Workout # _____

Exercise 1:	Exercise 2:	Exercise 3:	Exercise 4:
Total Reps:	Total Reps:	Total Reps:	Total Reps:
Weight:	Weight:	Weight:	Weight:

Tabata Tracker Date: _____ Tabata Workout # _____

Exercise 1:	Exercise 2:	Exercise 3:	Exercise 4:
Total Reps:	Total Reps:	Total Reps:	Total Reps:
Weight:	Weight:	Weight:	Weight:

Tabata Tracker Date: _____ Tabata Workout # _____

Exercise 1:	Exercise 2:	Exercise 3:	Exercise 4:
Total Reps:	Total Reps:	Total Reps:	Total Reps:
Weight:	Weight:	Weight:	Weight:

Tabata Tracker Date: _____ Tabata Workout # _____

Exercise 1:	Exercise 2:	Exercise 3:	Exercise 4:
Total Reps:	Total Reps:	Total Reps:	Total Reps:
Weight:	Weight:	Weight:	Weight:

Tabata Tracker Date: _____ Tabata Workout # _____

Exercise 1:	Exercise 2:	Exercise 3:	Exercise 4:
Total Reps:	Total Reps:	Total Reps:	Total Reps:
Weight:	Weight:	Weight:	Weight:

Tabata Tracker   Date: _____   Tabata Workout # _____

Exercise 1:	Exercise 2:	Exercise 3:	Exercise 4:
Total Reps:	Total Reps:	Total Reps:	Total Reps:
Weight:	Weight:	Weight:	Weight:

Tabata Tracker   Date: _____   Tabata Workout # _____

Exercise 1:	Exercise 2:	Exercise 3:	Exercise 4:
Total Reps:	Total Reps:	Total Reps:	Total Reps:
Weight:	Weight:	Weight:	Weight:

Tabata Tracker   Date: _____   Tabata Workout # _____

Exercise 1:	Exercise 2:	Exercise 3:	Exercise 4:
Total Reps:	Total Reps:	Total Reps:	Total Reps:
Weight:	Weight:	Weight:	Weight:

Tabata Tracker   Date: _____   Tabata Workout # _____

Exercise 1:	Exercise 2:	Exercise 3:	Exercise 4:
Total Reps:	Total Reps:	Total Reps:	Total Reps:
Weight:	Weight:	Weight:	Weight:

Tabata Tracker   Date: _____   Tabata Workout # _____

Exercise 1:	Exercise 2:	Exercise 3:	Exercise 4:
Total Reps:	Total Reps:	Total Reps:	Total Reps:
Weight:	Weight:	Weight:	Weight:

Tabata Tracker   Date: _____   Tabata Workout # _____

Exercise 1:	Exercise 2:	Exercise 3:	Exercise 4:
Total Reps:	Total Reps:	Total Reps:	Total Reps:
Weight:	Weight:	Weight:	Weight:

Tabata Tracker   Date: _____   Tabata Workout # _____

Exercise 1:	Exercise 2:	Exercise 3:	Exercise 4:
Total Reps:	Total Reps:	Total Reps:	Total Reps:
Weight:	Weight:	Weight:	Weight:

Tabata Tracker   Date: _____   Tabata Workout # _____

Exercise 1:	Exercise 2:	Exercise 3:	Exercise 4:
Total Reps:	Total Reps:	Total Reps:	Total Reps:
Weight:	Weight:	Weight:	Weight:

Tabata Tracker Date: _____ Tabata Workout # _____

Exercise 1:	Exercise 2:	Exercise 3:	Exercise 4:
Total Reps:	Total Reps:	Total Reps:	Total Reps:
Weight:	Weight:	Weight:	Weight:

Tabata Tracker Date: _____ Tabata Workout # _____

Exercise 1:	Exercise 2:	Exercise 3:	Exercise 4:
Total Reps:	Total Reps:	Total Reps:	Total Reps:
Weight:	Weight:	Weight:	Weight:

Tabata Tracker Date: _____ Tabata Workout # _____

Exercise 1:	Exercise 2:	Exercise 3:	Exercise 4:
Total Reps:	Total Reps:	Total Reps:	Total Reps:
Weight:	Weight:	Weight:	Weight:

Tabata Tracker Date: _____ Tabata Workout # _____

Exercise 1:	Exercise 2:	Exercise 3:	Exercise 4:
Total Reps:	Total Reps:	Total Reps:	Total Reps:
Weight:	Weight:	Weight:	Weight:

Tabata Tracker Date: _____ Tabata Workout # _____

Exercise 1:	Exercise 2:	Exercise 3:	Exercise 4:
Total Reps:	Total Reps:	Total Reps:	Total Reps:
Weight:	Weight:	Weight:	Weight:

Tabata Tracker Date: _____ Tabata Workout # _____

Exercise 1:	Exercise 2:	Exercise 3:	Exercise 4:
Total Reps:	Total Reps:	Total Reps:	Total Reps:
Weight:	Weight:	Weight:	Weight:

Tabata Tracker Date: _____ Tabata Workout # _____

Exercise 1:	Exercise 2:	Exercise 3:	Exercise 4:
Total Reps:	Total Reps:	Total Reps:	Total Reps:
Weight:	Weight:	Weight:	Weight:

Tabata Tracker Date: _____ Tabata Workout # _____

Exercise 1:	Exercise 2:	Exercise 3:	Exercise 4:
Total Reps:	Total Reps:	Total Reps:	Total Reps:
Weight:	Weight:	Weight:	Weight:

INDEX OF EXERCISES

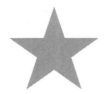

GOT QUESTIONS?
NEED ANSWERS?
GO TO:

GETFITNOW.COM
IT'S FITNESS 24/7

VIDEOS - WOROUTS- FORUMS
ONLINE STORE

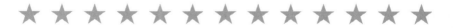